AF446842

Recent Results in Cancer Research

87

Founding Editor
P. Rentchnick, Geneva

Managing Editors
Ch. Herfarth, Heidelberg · H. J. Senn, St. Gallen

Associate Editors
M. Baum, London · C. von Essen, Villingen
V. Diehl, Hannover · W. Hitzig, Zürich
M. F. Rajewsky, Essen · C. Thomas, Marburg

F. F. Holmes

Aging and Cancer

With 58 Figures

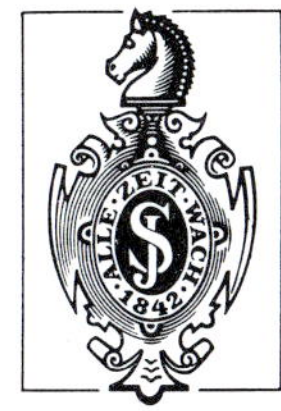

Springer-Verlag
Berlin Heidelberg New York Tokyo 1983

Frederick F. Holmes, M.D.

Hasinger Professor of Medicine and Gerontology
School of Medicine, The University of Kansas Medical Center,
Kansas City, KS 66103, USA

Sponsored by the Swiss League against Cancer

ISBN 3-540-12656-2 Springer-Verlag Berlin Heidelberg New York Tokyo
ISBN 0-387-12656-2 Springer-Verlag New York Heidelberg Berlin Tokyo

Library of Congress Cataloging in Publication Data. Main entry under title: Holmes, Frederick F., 1932– Aging and cancer. (Recent results in cancer research; 87) Includes index. 1. Geriatric oncology – Addresses, essays, lectures. I. Title. II. Series: Recent results in cancer research; v. 87. [DNLM: 1. Neoplasms. 2. Aging. W1 RE106P v. 87/QZ 200 H749a] RC281. A34H64 1983 618.97′6994 83-12511

Typesetting and printing: v. Starck'sche Druckereigesellschaft m.b.H., Wiesbaden
Binding: J. Schäffer OHG, Grünstadt
2125/3140–5 4 3 2 1 0

Dedicated to my parents, Margaret and Allan Holmes,
who have taught me the true meaning of graceful aging.

Contents

1 Introduction

The life of a human being is finite, and all humans age (see Fries 1980). It is difficult to separate the effects of disease on organs and tissues from those expected of aging. This is particularly true for vascular and degenerative processes, for which there are no clear boundaries between aging and disease. Morbidity and mortality from heart disease and stroke are probably due both to disease and to changes of aging. For cancer, the second leading cause of death in America, the situation is quite different; cancer is clearly a disease and is not a change expected with aging.

Cancer incidence increases almost logarithmically after age 40. In the United States about one-half of all cases of cancer are diagnosed after age 65, although those over 65 comprise less than one-eighth of the population. Thus, cancer is very much a disease of the elderly. There are at least two reasons for this: first, the prolonged exposure to cancer-inducing agents, and second, the waning power of immune defenses against cancer.

In treating cancer there are two possible objectives, cure or control. Some types of cancer are amenable to therapy for cure, that is, removal or destruction of the cancer so that it will never recur. Surgical removal of a lobe of a lung containing an early bronchial cancer or destruction by irradiation of an early cancer of the uterine cervix are salient examples. If cure is not possible, control becomes the objective of treatment. Hormonal therapy of breast cancer metastatic to the spine or chemotherapy of leukemia are examples of this latter objective. Control means partial destruction of the cancer or at least retardation of its growth. For both cure and control the best measure of success is prolongation of survival. Doctors treat patients one at a time; thus, the effectiveness of a particular treatment is evaluated one patient at a time. However, in order to establish that a method of cancer treatment is better than no treatment at all, or that one method of treatment is better than another, one must consider the experience of scores of patients to obtain statistical significance. Unfortunately this sort of elementary analysis of survival has not always been performed as often as it should have been in past years, which has led to well-meaning but misquided treatment strategies, the best example of which was the pre-1967 treatment of prostate cancer, which will be documented in Chapt 2.

Survival analysis for cancer patients can be done by a number of different methods, most of which seem to have been derived from the modification of actuarial analysis described by Berkson and Gage (1950). Comparisons can easily be made with survival curves for the population at large for various ages, making the excessive mortality from the disease being studied immediately apparent. An example is shown in Fig. 1, in which the 10-year survival of Kansans with chronic lymphocytic leukemia who were aged 65–74 at diagnosis (average age 69 years) is compared with the 10-year survival of 69-year-olds in Kansas from life tables derived from the 1970 census (Greville 1975).

Cancer is not a disease but a collection of diseases. Like the word "infection", that can describe both a boil and meningitis, which are vastly different in their import for the sufferer, cancer is a broad term. There are many varieties of cancer, perhaps even more than varieties of infection. The most elementary division is by site of origin of the cancer, quite specific for each cancer and, thus, for each patient. Site denotes the organ or tissue where the cancer first developed and is the major determinant of the behavior of that

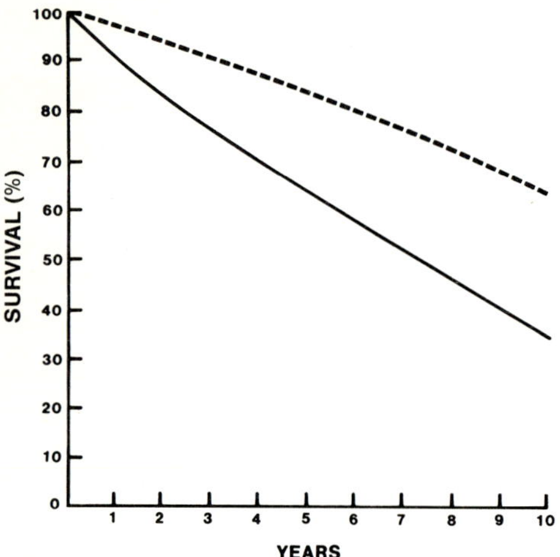

Fig. 1.1. Survival with chronic lymphocytic leukemia, diagnosed at ages 65–74 (*solid line*), vs 10-year survival of 69-year-olds (*broken line*)

cancer in a particular patient as long as it persists. Some common sites are breast, colon, brain, pancreas, and thyroid. As with infection, the impact on the patient is highly variable. Thyroid cancer is most often a very indolent disease, rarely the cause of death, and easily cured or controlled in most cases. By contrast, pancreatic cancer is almost always rapidly progressive, virtually never cured, and rarely controlled. Indeed the contrast between thyroid and pancreatic cancers may be even greater than the contrast between a boil and meningitis. No matter where a cancer spreads or metastasizes in a patient's body or how long the period from initial treatment to recurrence, the behavior of the cancer is mainly determined by its site of origin. There is a relationship of site to age as well. For example, thyroid and cervical cancers are most common in the young and middle-aged respectively, while prostate and rectal cancers are most common in the elderly.

For treatment planning and prognosis, the stage or extent of spread of a cancer at the time of diagnosis is a very important determination. There are many schemes for staging cancer; some are quite complex. However, the common denominator is a four-level system described in Table 1.1. After site of origin, stage at diagnosis is the most important determinant of survival.

In situ cancer is often called stage O. The best example is very early cancer of the uterine cervix detected by the Papanicolaou smear or Pap test. Only the outer surface of the cervix is involved and cure is almost certain. In about 25% of bronchial (lung) cancers the entire tumor appears to be within the lung with no spread to the chest wall, lymph nodes, or a distant place. This is local, or stage I, bronchial cancer. In breast cancer there may be growth of the cancer out of the breast tissue and into the overlying skin or spread by lymphatic vessels to the lymph nodes in the adjacent axilla. This is regional, or stage II, breast cancer. If the cancer has spread via the blood stream to a place or places quite distant from the site of origin, for example, breast cancer to bones of the spine, colonic cancer to the liver, or bronchial cancer to the brain, it is said to be stage III, or widespread or distant. There is no consistent relation of stage at diagnosis to age at diagnosis, though older people are more likely to have advanced cancers at diagnosis than are younger people (Holmes and Hearne 1981). Stage determined at diagnosis is the best approximation possible with the available data. Obviously, when relapse occurs after presumed curative treatment, many cancers originally staged as local are proved to have been distant.

Table 1. Stage of cancer at diagnosis

Stage	Extent of disease
In situ (0)	Confined to surface of site of origin
Local (I)	Confined to organ or tissue of origin
Regional (II)	Spread to area around organ of origin or to regional lymph nodes
Distant (III)	Spread to place(s) distant from site of origin

Histology is the microscopic appearance of the cells of a cancer and their organization or lack of it, and is yet another basis for classifying cancers. Histology is useful both in treatment planning and in prognosis, especially for leukemias and lymphomas. The site of origin of all leukemias is presumed to be the bone marrow, and one can consider leukemia equivalent to site designation such as thyroid, pancreas, and brain. Leukemia can be subdivided into many histologic types with vastly different prognoses. Acute monocytic leukemia and chronic lymphocytic leukemia are common in older people. Survival after diagnosis of the former is measured in weeks, and treatment is not often effective. Survival with the latter is measured in years, even without treatment.

Analyses of the duration of survival from time of diagnosis for cancer patients grouped by site and stage provide what may well be the best expositions of the natural histories of various types of cancers. This may sometimes be enhanced by separation according to sex, histology, and, very occasionally, race. However, this book will consider only site and stage.

Returning to the original considerations of age, we can appreciate that simple comparisons can be made between groups of cancer patients characterized by site and stage and age-matched segments of the general population. Since the expected duration of survival decreases with advancing age, it becomes apparent that age is a doubly critical factor in cancer. Increasing age is associated with ever-increasing cancer incidence but also with ever-decreasing life expectancy. The final consideration − one that cannot easily be quantified − is quality of life. Both cancer and its active treatment may cause pain and discomfort in addition to raising the specter of death. A child with cancer is usually in otherwise good health and, if cured, presumably has a life expectancy of many decades. Traditionally this is justification for very aggressive treatment aimed at cure and for acceptance of considerable morbidity and perhaps even some treatment-related mortality. However, in the older patient, who may well be frail and suffering from several chronic diseases, there is certainly much less justification for aggressive treatment that may cause much discomfort and that may even shorten a life that has but a few years remaining at best. Succinctly stated, in the elderly with cancer, we must be certain that we do not make the treatment worse than the disease. We must have a clear idea of the risks and benefits of various treatments and must be prepared to accept limited goals.

The following chapters in this book will consider cancers common to the elderly, each chapter addressing a particular site. Incidence rates in the first figure in each chapter are from the National Cancer Institute's *Surveillance Epidemiology, and End Results: Incidence and Mortality Data, 1973−1977* (Young et al. 1981). The remaining figures in each chapter are survival curves for the age-groups 65−74, 75−84, and 85−94 presented by stage at diagnosis (local, regional, and distant) during the periods 1950−1969 and 1970−1979 compared with the survival curves for these age groups in general in 1970. Data

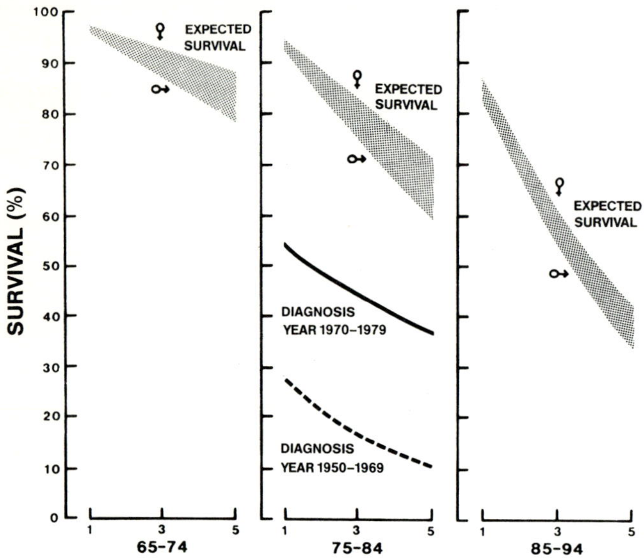

Fig. 1.2. Years survival by age and time groups according to site and stage

for the survival analyses are taken from computerized patient records of the Cancer Data Service and the Tumor Registry of the University of Kansas Medical Center. These data include more than 75,000 patients, of whom 37,907 were older than 64 years at time of diagnosis. Survival analysis is accomplished by the actuarial method of Berkson and Gage (1950) and is a measure of observed mortality expressed as percent survival for each year. Expected survival for each graph is calculated from Kansas Life Tables from the 1970 census (Greville 1975) using the average age for the group under consideration, a reasonable compromise for patients diagnosed in the 30-year time period 1950–1979. This is actually an estimate or approximation, but is appropriate for the data presented. Figure 1.2 shows the format for presentation of these survival data in subsequent chapters. When the term "significant" is used in the text, it means statistical significance at the 5% level.

References

Berkson J, Gage RP (1950) Calculation of survival rates for cancer. Proc Staff Meet Mayo Clinic 25:270–286

Fries JF (1980) Aging, natural death and the compression of morbidity. N Engl J Med 303:130–135

Greville TNE (1975) Kansas state life tables: 1969–1971, vol 2, no 17. National Center for Health Statistics, Washington DC (DHEW publication no 75-1151)

Holmes FF, Hearne EM (1981) Cancer stage-to-age relationship. J Am Geriatr Soc 29:55–57

Young JL, Percy CL, Asire AJ (1981) Surveillance, epidemiology and end-results: incidence and mortality data 1973–1977. Nat Cancer Inst Monogr 57 (NIH publication no 81-2330)

2 Prostate

The most prevalent cancer affecting elderly men in the United States originates in the prostate gland. With average age at diagnosis slightly exceeding 72 years, it is the quintessential cancer of old age. As shown in Fig. 2.1, incidence increases inexorably with age, reaching 344 per year per 100,000 of the 85-plus age-group. If annual incidence is expressed per 100,000 men of that age-group, it is 1,061 per 100,000.

Prostate cancer usually presents insidiously. The most common symptom is difficulty with urination from obstruction of the outlet from the bladder. The common symptoms of difficulty initiating urination and small urinary stream are also the presenting symptoms of benign prostatic hypertrophy, which many believe to be nearly universal among elderly American men. Prostate cancer is often diagnosed fortuitously. A hard nodule of cancer in the prostate may be palpated during examination of the rectum. Not infrequently, a small focus of early carcinoma or carcinoma in situ is found by an alert pathologist in the "chips" of prostatic tissue removed at transurethral resection for benign prostatic hypertrophy. On the other hand, every physician who sees elderly men as patients can remember men complaining of arthritis which in reality was bone pain from widespread bone metastases of prostate cancer, and men complaining of weakness and tiredness who proved to be anemic due to extensive replacement of their bone marrow with metastatic prostate cancer.

There are marked differences in the incidence of prostate cancer when one considers men from disparate groups. In America, prostate cancer is more common in black men than white men. Oriental men have an incidence rate much lower than that for white men. In

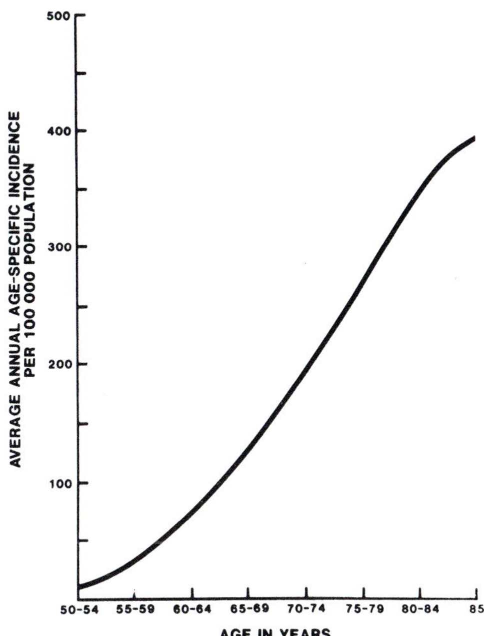

Fig. 2.1. Incidence of prostate cancer in USA 1973–1977

spite of these differences there is no real understanding at all of the cause or causes of prostate cancer.

There are two landmarks in the history of prostate cancer treatment. In 1966 Charles Huggins was awarded the Nobel Prize in Medicine for his 1941 description of the effects of castration and estrogens on prostate cancer and the implied benefits to patients (Huggins and Hodges 1941). Arduino et al. (1967) presented data from the first controlled trial for treatments for prostate cancer. Arduino and his associates established quite conclusively that there was no difference in duration of survival in respect of treatment. They proscribed castration for reasons other than symptom relief in advanced disease and noted, "what estrogen treatment wins from the cancer, it more than loses to other causes of death". Chemotherapy in prostate cancer has been an utter disappointment with no clear survival advantage demonstrated to date (Torti and Carter 1980). The most useful form of treatment in respect of prolonging survival has been radiation, particularly interstitial radiation, a fact long known but not sufficiently appreciated.

Local

During the period 1950—1979 there has been no significant improvement in survival for prostate cancer staged as local at diagnosis, as depicted in Fig. 2.2. Its contribution to mortality for the three age-groups lessens until it is inconsequential in the group of patients, 85—94 years old at time of diagnosis. The majority of these patients are treated surgically, with radiation of various sorts being used more frequently in recent years. The survival curves in Fig. 2.2 show quite clearly that prostate cancer of this stage is usually a very indolent disease. There is no meaning in the idea of a 5-year cure. In fact, many believe that this disease is rarely if ever cured at any stage. At least in the age-groups presented here there is no justification for mutilation or radical treatment as an attempt to cure a few patients.

Just about half of these patients die with evidence of persistence of their prostate cancer, and half have no obvious evidence of this disease at death. Given the survival experience

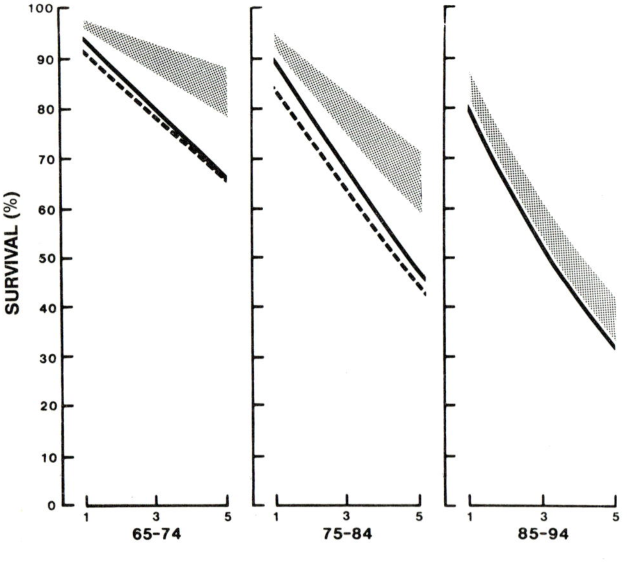

Fig. 2.2. Years survival by age and time groups for locally confined prostate cancer

shown in Fig. 2.2, the indolence of the disease generally, and the fact that it is probably not curable, the most sensible disease management strategy would seem to be control of disease manifestations. This would include early identification of disease recurrence or progression.

Regional

In several respects, regionally spread prostate cancer is quite a different disease than that which is locally confined. Though still often an indolent disease, this stage shortens life considerably and progresses more rapidly. Cure of disease is really not even a remote possibility. Excessive mortality is noted even after 5 years in all but the oldest age-group. However, there is good news to be derived from the 30-year data for this stage of prostate cancer. There is a statistically significant increase in survival at 1, 2, and 4 years for the 65−74 age group; at 1 and 2 years for the 75−84 age-group; and at 5 years for the 85−94 age-group. There are at least two reasons for this: In the 1970s estrogen was used less frequently and, when used, in much smaller amounts than in the 1950s and 1960s; external beam and interstitial radiation have been more extensively used in recent years.
The great irony of prostate cancer treatment is clearly shown in the 85−94 age-group (Figs. 2, 3). Survival in the 1970s nearly equals that of the general age-matched male population, a vast improvement over the period 1950−1969. In fact, there is little ground left to gain at this age. Regionally spread prostate cancer can be said to have minimal influence on mortality in this group of the old, now that estrogen treatment has been appropriately reduced.
Curves from the two younger age groups show that there is still excessive mortality that might be reduced, although not by much. The best treatment strategy seems to be an aggressive effort to control the cancer in the pelvis at the time of diagnosis, with early identification of disease progression or recurrence and appropriate control measures then applied. Given the limits of surgery in this regard and the futility of chemotherapy as presently practiced in this disease, a major role is suggested for radiotherapy.

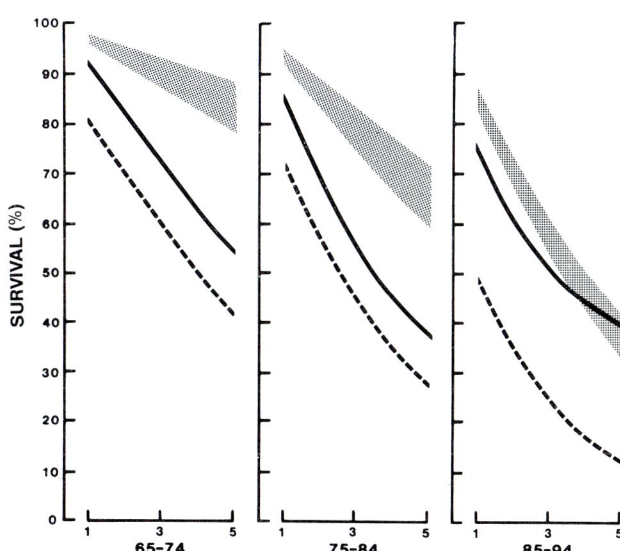

Fig. 2.3. Years survival by age and time groups for regionally spread prostate cancer

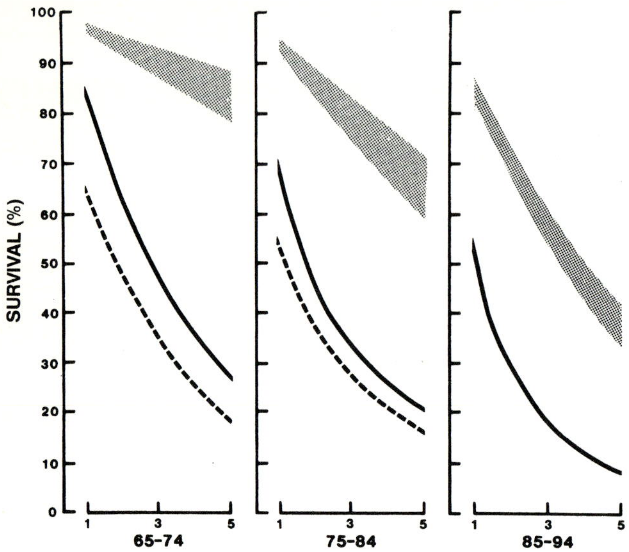

Fig. 2.4. Years survival by age and time groups for distantly spread prostate cancer

Distant

Prostate cancer widespread at diagnosis is not easily treated; it is a systemic disease and taxes the skill of any physician. Because extensive bone metastases are the rule at this stage, the patient is often disabled by bone pain. The curves in Fig. 2.4 show improved survival during the 30 years of the study, but this is significant only at 1 year in the 65−74 age group. Modification of estrogen doses is probably as responsible for this modest improvement as any other factor. Of course, virtually all patients with this stage of disease die with the disease, but not always of it.

Perhaps the remarkable feature about this stage is that 5-year survival is 20%−25% something not seen in other cancers widespread at diagnosis, again a testimony to the indolence of the disease in many cases. However, its mortality is high, even in the oldest age group.

Surgery and radiation have very limited roles to play at this stage of the disease. This group of patients needs effective systemic therapy, probably chemotherapy or something closely akin to it. Unfortunately, nothing appropriate and effective is presently available. However, with control of symptoms, particularly bone pain, it is remarkable how many men with this stage of disease may have years of comfortable and useful life.

References

Arduino LJ, Bailar JC, The Veteran's Administration Cooperative Urological Research Group (1967) Carcinoma of the prostate: treatment comparisons. J Urol 98: 516−522
Huggins C, Hodges CV (1941) The effect of castration, of estrogen and of androgen injection on serum phosphatases in metastatic carcinoma of the prostate. Cancer Res 1: 293−297
Torti FM, Carter SK (1980) The chemotherapy of prostatic adenocarcinoma. Ann Intern Med 92: 681−689

3 Breast

Probably no cancer causes more human suffering and grief or has received more attention in recent years than breast cancer. Though breast cancer is the most common cause of death for middle-aged women in America, it is not often appreciated that the incidence climbs steadily into old age, as shown in Fig. 3.1. Indeed, the chance that an 85-year-old woman will develop breast cancer is just about double that for a 50-year-old woman in America. Although the causes of breast cancer are not known, there is a fairly clear understanding of risk factors, such as early menarche, late menopause, nulliparity, or late primiparity, to name only a few. The common denominator seems to be alteration of estrogen metabolism attendant on these several factors (Dickinson et al. 1974). An unrelated risk factor is radiation to the breast after puberty, which is very ironic because mammography itself delivers radiation to the breast. Quite beyond this, mammography is especially efficient in the older breast, which has a greater contrast between fat and breast tissue per se (Strax 1976; Swartz and Reichling 1977).

The controversies about treatment of breast cancer are several, and are not completely resolved by any means. Halstead (1894) described radical mastectomy in 50 patients, which remained the essentially unquestioned treatment for breast cancer until challenged by Crile (1974). It is still not certain what is the best operation for breast cancer. Beyond this there is considerable feeling that radiation of early breast cancer may be just as good treatment as surgery (Mansfield 1976). Finally, to complete the confusion, the utility of chemotherapy as adjuvant treatment following surgery to prevent recurrence is now fairly well

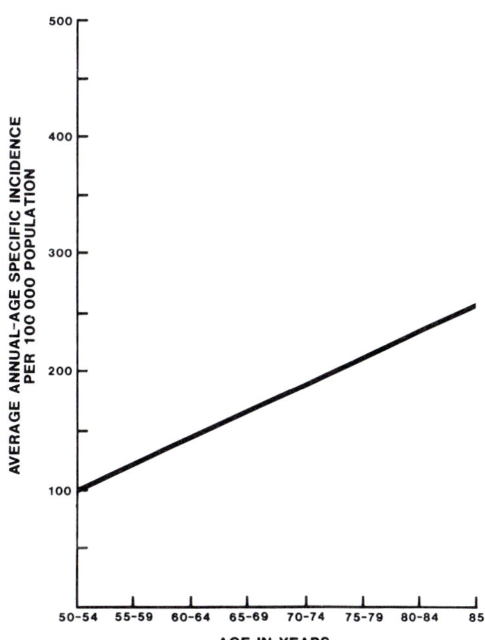

Fig. 3.1. Incidence of breast cancer in USA 1973–1977

established. That adjuvant chemotherapy will also extend life is not completely established. A question of methodology in the major early study has led to some confusion about whether or not elderly women benefit from adjuvant chemotherapy as much as do middle-aged women, and this uncertainty is unfortunate (Bonadonna 1979).

It is difficult to answer definitely questions about breast cancer because it is a capricious disease, chronic for some women and acute for others. Even cursory inspection of survival curves shows that 5-year disease-free survival does not mean cure, as it does in so many kinds of cancer. In fact, the record for the interval from initial treatment for cure to recurrence is 50 years with intervals of 20 years or so sufficiently common that they are not reported (Sutton 1960).

All of these factors and controversies have special relevance for older women with breast cancer. Minimal rather than extensive and mutilating surgery seems quite appropriate for the elderly. Long-term complications of radiation and chemotherapy have little relevance in older patients. Thus, if radiation of limited breast cancer is as good as surgery, it is an excellent choice for the elderly woman. When life expectancy is measured in years rather than in decades, early recurrence of breast cancer becomes much more important than late recurrence. Adjuvant chemotherapy seems to be particularly efficacious for elderly women if its benefits are clearly established and if accompanying discomfort and inconvenience are less than the disability of recurrence (Begg et al. 1980).

Even beyond these considerations is the fact that breast cancer as a chronic disease may be just one more chronic disease for an elderly woman who already has several chronic diseases which are not curable. Thus, control and management become primary strategies, with a valiant attempt at cure often much less appropriate.

Local

Survival with cancer confined to the breast at diagnosis is surprisingly good. In viewing Fig. 3.2 one must remember to compare the two survival curves with the top margin of the

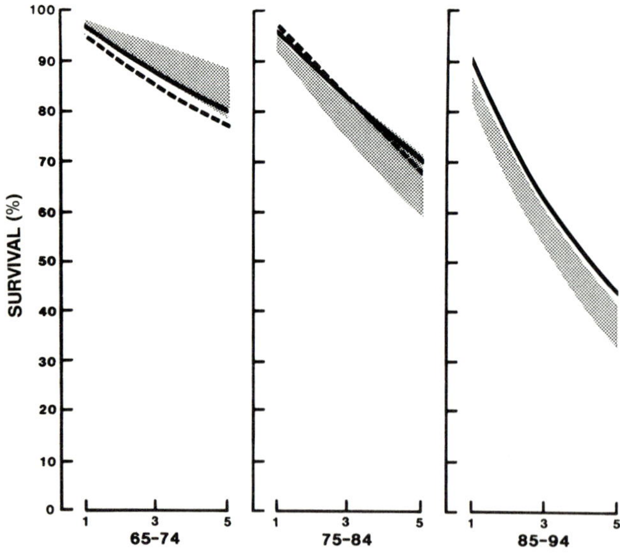

Fig. 3.2. Years survival by age and time groups for locally confined breast cancer

gray area. Most women in this stage of disease are cured by initial treatment, usually surgery. Unfortunately, these data can not be used to answer the questions of how much surgery is enough or whether radiation is as good as surgery in treating this stage of disease.

Figure 3.2 shows no significant or even apparent increase in survival in the 30 years of this study. Excessive mortality, in the youngest age-group particularly, is due to the early progression of distantly spread disease not detected at the time of diagnosis, and to late recurrence. Interestingly, breast cancer per se exerts little influence on mortality in the two older age-groups, most deaths being from other causes, though early progression is a factor of importance and worth recognition.

The challenge in this stage of disease is to prevent or at least delay early progression of distantly spread, undetected disease. Chemotherapy adjuvant to potentially curative therapy has been proposed as the appropriate strategy. Unfortunately, one has to accept the fact that most women so treated are already cured and are, thus, needlessly exposed to the dangers and discomforts of chemotherapy. In the data for the 1950–1969 period there were 212 women with locally confined breast cancer at diagnosis who were between 65 and 74 years of age. Of these, 65 (30.7%) died with breast cancer; 15 (7.1%) of the deaths occurred 10 or more years after diagnosis. A woman in the 65–74 age-group has, on the average, a life expectancy of 15 years. She has much to gain if adjuvant chemotherapy works. At least in regionally spread disease it seems to delay early disease progression and perhaps increases survival duration. The long-term complications of adjuvant chemotherapy have yet to be defined, but may well include increased risk of second cancers, particularly acute leukemia. Whether or not adjuvant chemotherapy will alter patterns of later recurrence of breast cancer will take some years to learn. This is an important factor for women in the 65–74 age-group, though of relatively little importance for those in the two older age-groups.

Analysis of this stage of disease could perhaps best be summed up by stating that locally confined breast cancer is a disease which is usually and easily cured for most women, but is likely to become chronic for those not cured.

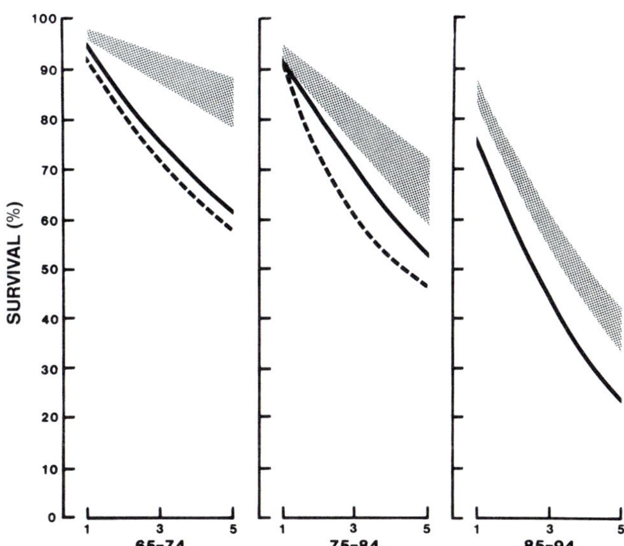

Fig. 3.3. Years survival by age and time groups for regionally spread breast cancer

Regional

Regional spread of this disease means progression of disease into lymphatic tissue usually either in the axilla or in the skin overlying the breast. Figure 3.3 shows apparent modest improvement in survival over the 30 years of this study, but this is not statistically significant. Excessive mortality from breast cancer is apparent in all three age-groups. More than half of the women with breast cancer in this stage at diagnosis eventually die with or of their disease, as data from the 1950−1969 period prove (115 of 216 dead with disease, 32 dead more than 5 years after diagnosis). Thus, a sizable minority of women with breast cancer at this stage are probably cured, but for most it is a chronic disease.
For all age-groups in this study prevention or delay of early progression of disease is the most important goal. Late recurrence is still of some importance, particularly for the 65−74 age-group, but its prevention or further delay is much less important than that of earlier progression. Thus, chemotherapy adjuvant to initial treatment assumes a high order of importance.

Distant

All women with this stage of breast cancer at time of diagnosis die of or with their disease. Figure 3.4 shows a high mortality for all three age groups. At least in the 65−74 age-group, survival is significantly increased at 1, 2, and 3 years. The only plausible explanation for this is the efficacy of multiagent chemotherapy protocols used extensively during the 1970s. It may also be true for the two older groups, but the number of cases in the 1950−1969 time period was too small for meaningful analysis in this study.
Again, it is surprising that for some women this is a chronic disease, even when diagnosed at this advanced stage. Actuarial uncorrected 5-year survival is 23.3% in the 65−74 age-group in the 1970s. Occasionally, chemotherapy and/or hormone therapy produce fairly long periods of apparent disease-free remission, even at this stage. The challenge for

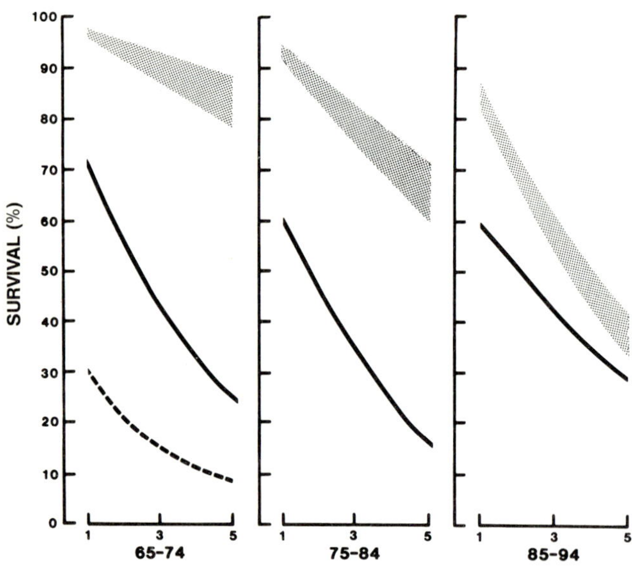

Fig. 3.4. Years survival by age and time groups for distantly spread breast cancer

management of this stage of breast cancer is control of disease principally by systemic therapy. Past successes seem to indicate that more effective multi-agent protocols can be devised.

References

Begg CB, Cohen JL, Ellerton J (1980) Are the elderly predisposed to toxicity from cancer chemotherapy? Cancer Clin Trial 3:369–374

Bonadonna G (1979) Adjuvant chemotherapy for breast cancer. Lancet 1:1397

Crile G Jr (1974) Management of breast cancer: limited mastectomy. JAMA 230:95–98

Dickinson LE, MacMahon B, Cole P, Brown JB (1974) Estrogen profiles of oriental and caucasian women in Hawaii. N Engl J Med 291:1211–1213

Halsted WS (1894) The results of operations for the cure of cancer of the breast performed at Johns Hopkins Hospital from June 1889 to January 1894. Ann Surg 20:497–555

Mansfield CM (1976) Early breast cancer, its history and results of treatment. Karger, New York (Experimental biology and medicine, vol 5)

Strax P (1976) Results of mass screening for breast cancer in 50,000 examinations. Cancer 37:30–35

Sutton M (1960) Late recurrence of carcinoma of the breast. Br Med J 1:1132–1134

Swartz HM, Reichling BA (1977) The risks of mammograms. JAMA 236:955–966

4 Bronchus

The great self-induced cancer of our time, of course, is lung or, more accurately identified in the anatomic sense, bronchial cancer. The link with cigarette smoking is sufficiently certain to regard it as a cause of lung cancer. Interestingly, the incidence of lung cancer in America is not the world's highest; America lags behind many western European countries in this regard (Waterhouse et al. 1976). At one time lung cancer was essentially a disease of men, with an 8 : 1 male-to-female ratio. However, this is now changing and the incidence of lung cancer is rising sharply in America, probably mostly related to the increasing popularity of cigarette smoking among women in recent decades. It is even possible that at some future time lung cancer will become more common in women than in men, if the present trend of more teenage girls smoking than teenage boys continues and this ratio persists throughout life (Meigs 1977; National Cancer Institute and American Cancer Society 1977).

In Fig. 4.1 we see that the incidence of bronchial cancer reaches its apex in the seventies and then declines rather rapidly in the eighties. Of the possible reasons for this, two seem most plausible. First, it may be that fewer people in their eighties today have ever smoked than have those of the present population between the ages 70 and 79. Perhaps a more likely possibility is that the effects of cigarette smoking as a cause of lung cancer are a spent force in the very elderly. Those who were susceptible to the damaging effects of cigarette smoking by way of death from heart attack, emphysema, and lung cancer are gone by age 80 or so. There are some folks who survive into the eighties after a life of heavy smoking, but these people are not numerous.

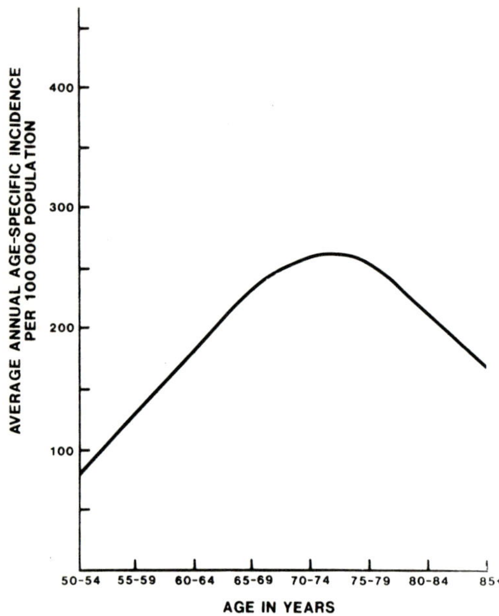

Fig. 4.1. Incidence of bronchial cancer in USA 1973–1977

Lung cancer is rarely a chronic disease in the sense that prostate or breast cancer so often is. Survival free of disease for even 3 years after diagnosis and surgical treatment with curative intent usually means cure. The great tragedy of lung cancer is that few are indeed cured. There is a useful generalization about lung cancer that puts this into sharp focus. For every 100 patients diagnosed as having lung cancer, only 50 are candidates for consideration of curative (surgical) treatment. The other 50 either have regional or widespread disease beyond the scope of surgical resection or are so disabled from other lung disease, usually emphysema, as to prohibit consideration of a chest operation or removal of any lung tissue. Of the 50 who undergo surgery, 25 are found to have cancer sufficiently widespread within the chest to preclude an attempt at curative resection of lung tissue. Of the 25 who have potentially curative surgery, five are alive 5 years later. This makes for a cure rate of about 5%. The average survival for all lung cancer patients is well under 1 year, both mean and median.

There is a curious paradox in the elderly patient with lung cancer. In distinction to virtually all other sites of cancer, there is an inverse relationship between age and stage; that is, the older patient is more likely to have locally confined lung cancer than the younger patient (Holmes and Hearne 1981). Thus, on this basis alone, more older patients than younger ones might be considered candidates for thoracotomy. However, thoracotomy with resection of the lung is very major surgery at any age. Coexistent heart disease, emphysema, and the basic lung and thorax changes with aging make most chest surgeons think long and hard before they operate on those over 70.

Local

Bronchial cancer is not a chronic disease; it is an acute disease. Even in those with disease locally confined at diagnosis just about half are dead after 1 year. Five-year survival almost always means cure at any age. Late recurrence of dormant disease is virtually unknown. As shown in Fig. 4.2, survival is poor in all three groups of elderly patients. There is no change, either apparent or significant, during the 30 years of this study. At the present time

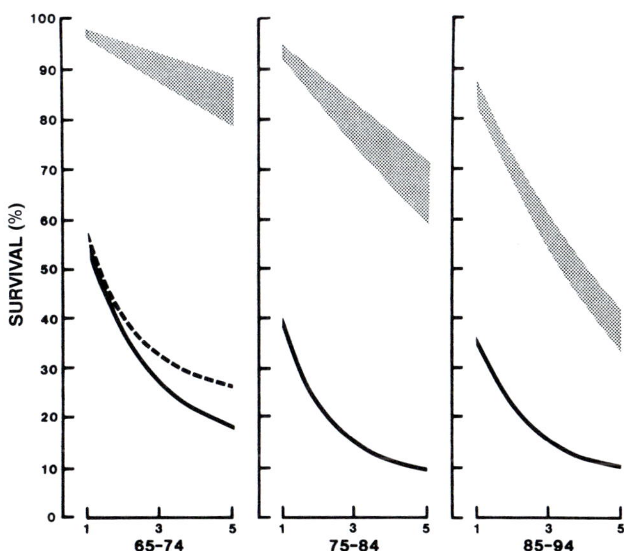

Fig. 4.2. Years survival by age and time groups for locally confined bronchial cancer

cure is possible only with surgery. Various schemes for adjuvant immunotherapy, radiotherapy, and chemotherapy have consistently failed to improve survival except in small-cell carcinoma (Einhorn et al. 1976). Lung cancer is so common and so rapidly progressive, and survival so poor, that it has been the ideal kind of cancer for such trials. In one such controlled trial the group with the longest survival was composed of patients who were offered potentially curative surgery but refused operation. Another study demonstrated − to the consternation of some − best survival in patients who had pleural infection as a complication of chest surgery for lung cancer (Ruckeschel et al. 1972). The elderly patient with lung cancer deserves a candid description of the nature of the disease and its treatment. For the elderly patient with locally confined disease who also has good cardiopulmonary function the chance of survival is one in five at best.

Actually, surgical experience in bronchial cancer in the elderly is considerable. In larger series reported in the literature the operative mortality is acceptable, and the cure rates are essentially the same as for younger patients. However, this presumes a patient who has sufficiently good heart and lung function to permit thoracotomy (Wellington and Lynn 1966; Kirsh et al. 1976).

A recent paper by Cox et al. (1980) suggests that irradiation may be very effective therapy for inoperable bronchial cancer in patients who are otherwise generally well. They report that some patients may actually have been cured by this treatment.

Regional

The one ray of hope in lung cancer seems to be the fact that survival improved at 1 and 2 years when the 1950−1969 and the 1970−1979 time periods are compared. This is shown in Fig. 4.3 for the 65−74 age-group as significant at 1 and 2 years and apparent at 3 years. This increase in survival is apparent in the 75−84 age-group but not significant, perhaps because the number of patients is smaller. There were not sufficient patients to provide survival curves for the oldest age-group. The fact that the survival increase is lost at 4 and 5 years suggests retardation of the disease or improved control, not an increased cure rate.

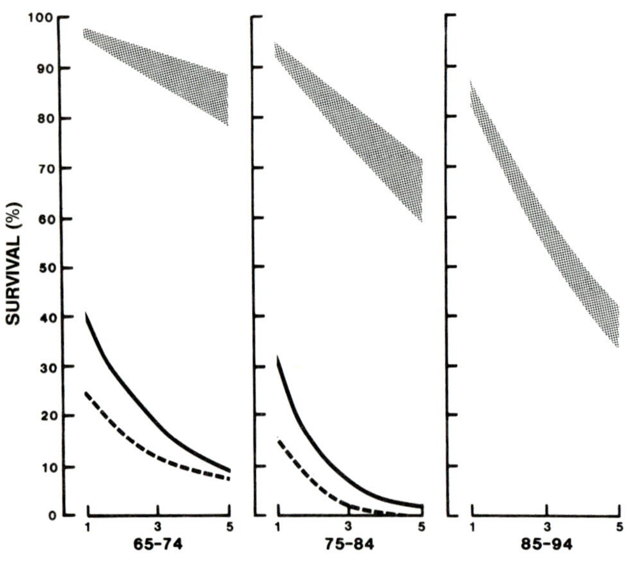

Fig. 4.3. Years survival by age and time groups for regionally spread bronchial cancer

It is important to note that from 2%–3% of patients are cured at this stage, and this percentage has not changed with the years. The reasons for this improvement in short-term survival are not clear. Decrease in operative mortality, control of the primary tumor, control of infection, and temporary benefit of radiotherapy all seem to be possibilities. Except with the histologic group of small cell cancers, there is no reason to believe that chemotherapy has contributed much to this improvement.

Distant

Most patients diagnosed at this stage die of their disease, and all die with it. Though systemic chemotherapy does considerably improve survival in small cell histology, it is probably rarely if ever curative. In this stage more than 80% are dead at 1 year. Though there is an apparent small increase in survival in the 65–74 and 75–84 age-groups, this increase is not significant.

Lung cancer metastasizes early and widely, brain metastases being almost certain if the patient lives long enough. Most chemotherapeutic agents do not cross the blood-brain barrier so there is, at least at present, an absolute limit to the potential of chemotherapy. Quite apart from this, there have been many single- and multiple-agent chemotherapy trials in this stage of the disease. None have changed the course of the disease to an appreciable extent, and many have extracted a considerable toll in morbidity and misery for the patient, who is often in the preterminal phase of his illness at this point.

Radiotherapy is of palliative benefit for bone pain at this stage and can be given in short courses to great benefit. It must be admitted that at present there is little more to offer the patient than palliation.

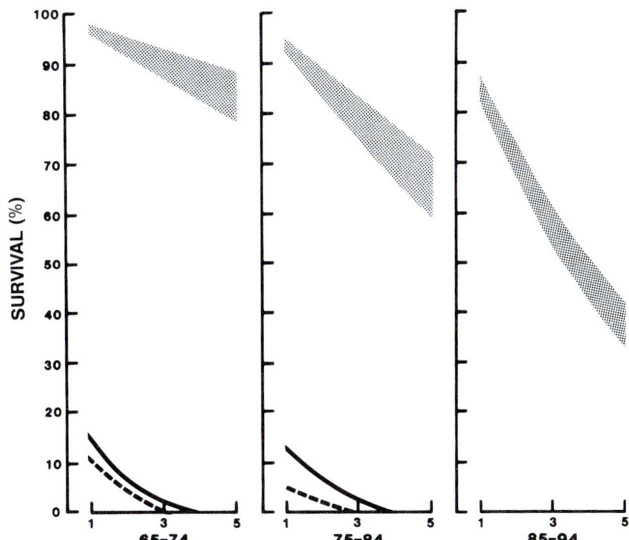

Fig. 4.4. Years survival by age and time groups for distantly spread bronchial cancer

References

Cox JD, Komaki R, Eierst DR (1980) Irradiation for inoperable carcinoma of the lung and high performance status. JAMA 244: 1931–1933

Einhorn LH, Fee WH, Farber MO, Linvingston RB, Gottlieb JA (1976) Improved chemotherapy for small-cell undifferentiated lung cancer. JAMA 235: 1225–1229

Holmes FF, Hearne EM (1981) Cancer stage-to-age relationship: implications for cancer screening in the elderly. J Am Geriatr Soc 29: 55–57

Kirsh MM, Rotman H, Bove E, Argenta L, Cimmino V, Tashian J, Ferguson P, Sloan H (1976) Major pulmonary resection for bronchogenic carcinoma in the elderly. Ann Thorac Surg 22: 369–373

Meigs JW (1977) Epidemic lung cancer in women. JAMA 238: 1055

National Cancer Institute and American Cancer Society (1977) Cigarette smoking among teenagers and young women. United States Public Health Service, Bethesda (DHEW publication no (NIH) 77-1208)

Ruckdeschel JC, Codish SD, Stranahan A, McKneally MF (1972) Postoperative empyema improves survival in lung cancer. N Engl J Med 287: 1013–1017

Waterhouse J, Muir C, Correa P, Powell J (1976) Cancer incidence in five continents, vol 3. International Agency for Research on Cancer, Lyon (IARC scientific publications no 15)

Wellington JL, Lynn RB (1966) Thoracic surgery in the elderly. Can Med Assoc J 95: 252–256

5 Stomach

For unknown reasons the incidence of stomach cancer in America has declined markedly in the 50 years from 1930 to 1980. This decrease is on the order of fourfold. No credit is due the medical profession for this remarkable salutary change in what is one of the worst kinds of cancer a person may suffer. As there is no clear understanding of the cause, it is not possible to understand the improvement. While it is thought that consumption of smoked fish may be related to stomach cancer — incidence is high in Japan and Iceland — there are obviously other operative factors. It does seem likely that environmental factors are most important in initiation of this cancer and that America's consumption of cleaner water and food may be important in its declining incidence. This decreasing incidence certainly diminishes ones fears about food additives (Silverberg 1982; Haenszel and Correa 1975).

Figure 5.1 shows stomach cancer to be a disease of older people. The incidence increases by a factor of almost 10 from age 50 to 85+. There is a male predominence of about two to one for which there is no clear explanation. Few cases are diagnosed as truly locally confined and the 5-year survival rate for all cases has been in the neighborhood of 5% for many years. Though few survive 5 years with this disease, those who do are almost always cured; surgical resection of the entire cancer offers the only hope. Stomach cancer is largely resistant to radiation treatment and chemotherapy results have been uniformly disappointing; only limited palliation seems possible with these agents (Macdonald et al. 1980). Occasionally lymphoma is primary to the stomach, and this disease may be cured or

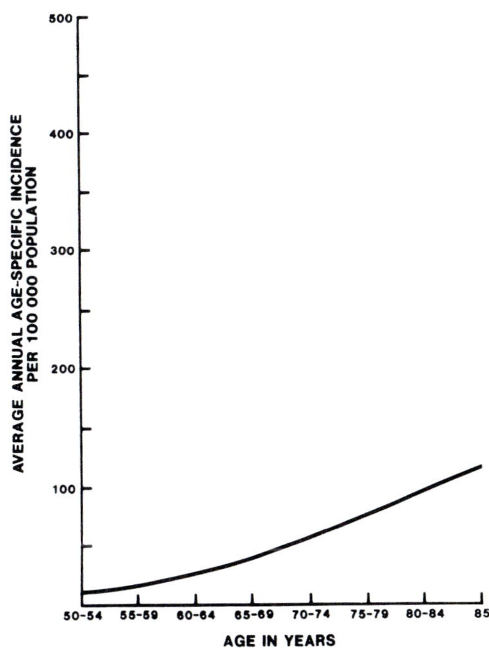

Fig. 5.1. Incidence of stomach cancer in USA 1973–1977

controlled for long periods, in contrast to the very great majority which are carcinomas.

Anorexia, weight loss, and anemia are common symptoms of stomach cancer in the elderly. Diagnosis by X-ray and endoscopy is relatively straightforward. Choice of treatment usually is choice of palliation. This is a great challenge when the patient is elderly and debilitated.

Local

When stomach cancer is truly locally confined the chance for cure is surprisingly good regardless of age, as shown in Fig. 5.2. Five-year survival almost always means cure. Long persistence or late recurrence of this disease are unknown. It is unfortunate that there was an insufficient number of cases to make meaningful survival curves for the early time period and for the oldest age-group. Cure is possible only with radical surgery, and there is little reason to believe that surgical techniques have really improved in the past 30 years, so survival rates are probably not better.

Vastly improved techniques and instruments for endoscopy have opened the way for earlier diagnosis of this disease. Interestingly, in the 1950–1969 time period only 6.1% of cases were staged as local at diagnosis while 20.1% were staged as local in the 1970–1979 period. It would seem quite appropriate to utilize endoscopy liberally when stomach cancer is a consideration, particularly in the elderly (Fielding et al. 1980).

Adjuvant radiotherapy and chemotherapy have not proved very useful in this disease at this stage, and the relatively rapid course of the disease makes evaluation of such regimens fairly easy.

Thus, though this is a cancer of declining incidence, it is of considerable importance in the elderly and will probably remain so. It might even be regarded as sufficiently common, and cure rates for early disease good enough, to consider screening programs for the elderly.

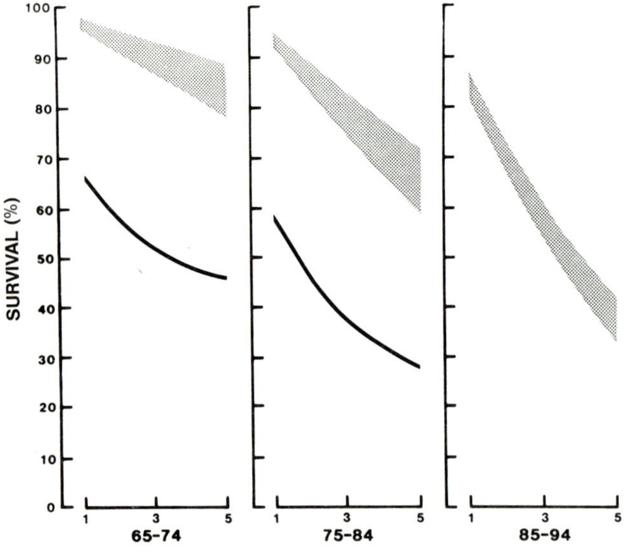

Fig. 5.2. Years survival by age and time groups for locally confined stomach cancer

Regional

More patients present with their disease at this stage than at any other. Spread to regional lymph nodes and into adjacent organs probably occurs before symptoms of the disease appear for the majority of patients. Though cure by radical surgery is still possible, it is a relative rarity. Figure 5.3 shows a clear trend toward improvement in survival in the two time periods, which is significant in the 75−84 age-group at 1 year in spite of the relatively small number of patients. This most surely represents temporary control or retardation of disease rather than an increase in the miniscule cure rate at this stage, or earlier diagnosis even within the regionally spread stage. The notorious resistance of this cancer to radiotherapy and chemotherapy makes the latter possibility most likely.

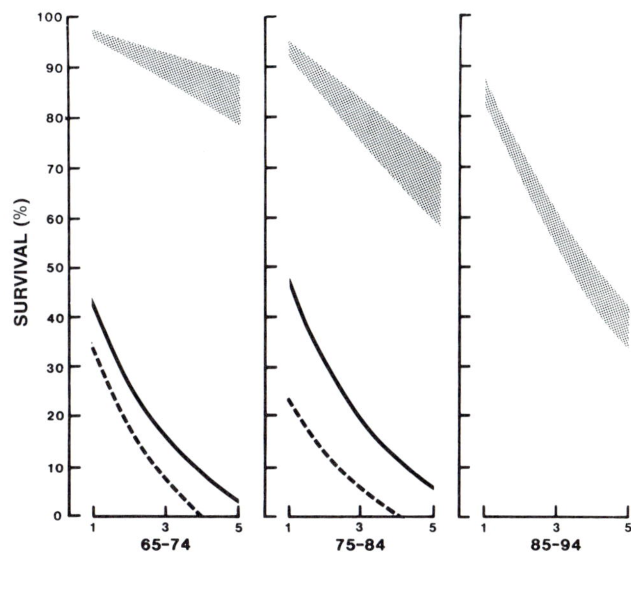

Fig. 5.3. Years survival by age and time groups for regionally spread stomach cancer

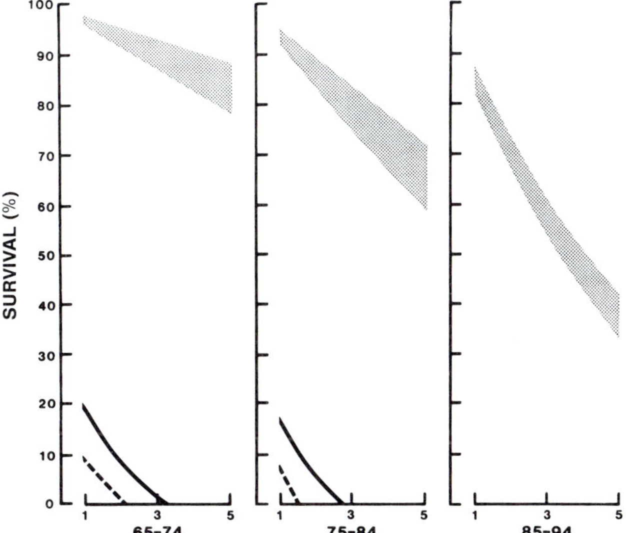

Fig. 5.4. Years survival by age and time groups for distantly spread stomach cancer

The challenge to the physician is palliation and comfort for the older patient with stomach cancer at this stage. Obviously, it is appropriate to continue to search for means of controlling the growth rate of this cancer but, particularly in the elderly patient, this should not be done in ways that add to the misery of an already miserable illness.

Distant

All patients die of or with their disease at this stage. Though there is an apparent small increase in survival in the 65–74 and 75–84 age-groups between the two time periods this is not, with the numbers available, significant (Fig. 5.4). It seems that only chemotherapy can be expected to alter this dismal picture. Virtually all of these patients have extensive metastases to their livers because of the geography of portal vein blood flow. Liver metastases are notoriously resistant to all modalities of treatment no matter what the site of the primary cancer. When the disease is diagnosed at this stage most patients can be considered terminally ill, and palliation is the challenge to the physician.

References

Fielding JWL, Ellis DJ, Jones BG, Paterson J, Powell DJ, Waterhouse JAH, Brookes VS (1980) Natural history of early gastric cancer: results of a 10-year survey. Br Med J 281: 965–967
Haenszel W, Correa P (1975) Developments in the epidemiology of stomach cancer over the past decade. Cancer Res 35: 3452–3459
Macdonald JS, Schein PS, Woolley PV, Smythe T, Ueno W, Hoth D, Smith F, Boiron M, Gisselbrecht C, Brunet R, Lagarde C (1980) 5-Fluorouracil, doxorubicin, and mitomycin (FAM) combination chemotherapy for advanced gastric cancer. Ann Intern Med 93: 533–536
Silverberg E (1982) Cancer statistics. CA 32: 15–42

6 Colon and Rectum

We often forget that colorectal carcinoma is the most common kind of visceral cancer in America and very much a disease of the elderly. It is more common than lung, breast, or prostate cancer. As shown in Fig. 6.1, the incidence at age 50−54 is 51.5 per 100,000 per year, more than doubling every decade until it is 451.1 at age 80−84. Colorectal cancer is equally common in men and women.

There seems to be every reason to believe that most colorectal cancers have a cause related to the environment, particularly the environment within the gut. The major question is, what are the environmental factors; surely there are at least several (Rhodes et al. 1977). The second question is related to the importance of benign precursor lesions, particularly the very common adenomatous polyp. One can read the classic paper of Castleman and Krickstein (1962) and decide that adenomatous polyps have little malignant potential, but the very practical paper of Gilbertsen and Nelms (1978) proves that the incidence of rectal cancer is markedly decreased when adenomatous polyps are periodically removed.

Recent years have seen appreciation of the fact that screening of large populations for occult blood in the stool is useful in detecting symptomless colorectal cancers. The procedure is cheap and simple but there are many false positives as well as false negatives, and thus problems with both sensitivity and specificity. However, the weight of medical opinion seems to favor such screening periodically, especially in the elderly (Sherlock et al. 1980). Surgical treatment of colorectal cancer evokes the thought of colostomy in the minds of most people. There is little challenge to the efficacy of this fairly radical surgery in

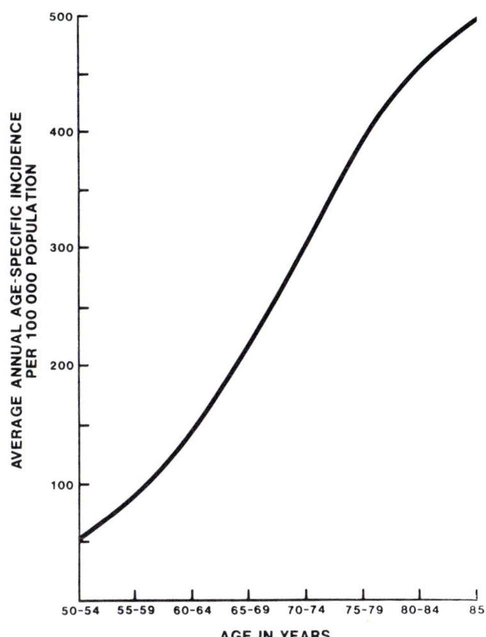

Fig. 6.1. Incidence of colon and rectum cancer in USA 1973−1977

contrast to radical mastectomy for breast cancer. Particularly in the frail elderly, however, there is good reason to consider other treatment techniques. More conservative surgery and radiation of the primary lesion are currently enjoying some popularity (Clarke et al. 1980; Miller and Allbritten 1976; Papillon 1975).

Local

When the cancer is truly locally confined at diagnosis, cure rates are good at any age. Figure 6.2 shows apparent small improvement in survival in the 1950−1979 period, but this is not statistically significant in spite of hundreds of cases for comparison. Though late recurrence or late mortality does occur in colorectal cancer, 5-year survival usually means cure. Patients with disease locally confined at diagnosis who die of their disease after apparently curative treatment are victims of systemically spread disease too small to detect at the time of diagnosis. The 1950−1969 data show that 30% of patients died with or of their disease.

Adjuvant chemotherapy and radiation therapy have not proved of sufficient efficacy to date to be widely used. Theoretically, this would seem to be a good situation for adjuvant chemotherapy. The unfortunate truth is that no single- or multi-agent chemotherapy regimen has gained more than limited acceptance (Li and Ross 1976).

Early detection of colorectal cancer seems to be the best strategy for increasing cure rates. If all colorectal cancers were found and treated in the local stage, the cure rate would be about 70%. Rectal cancer is usually diagnosed earlier than colonic cancer. A disquieting factor is that, though the incidence of colorectal cancer has remained fairly stable in America over recent decades, there is evidence that the incidence of rectal cancer is decreasing while that of right-side-of-colon cancer is increasing (Rhodes et al. 1977). This gives even greater credence to periodic screening of stools for occult blood and even to liberal use of barium enema X-ray examinations, particularly in the elderly, until a more specific screening test is developed.

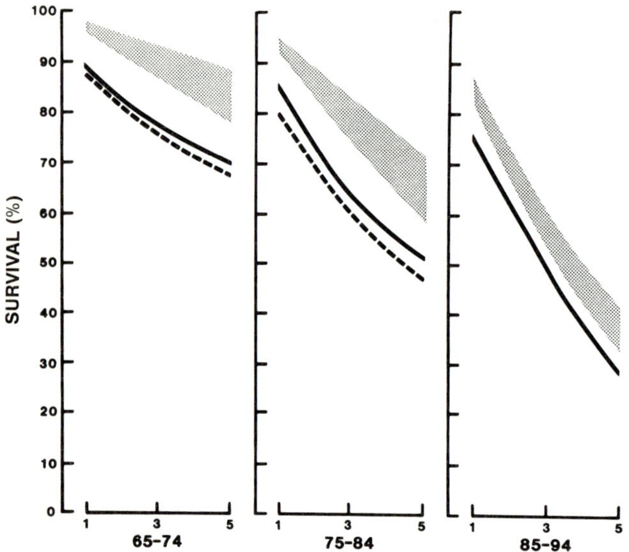

Fig. 6.2. Years survival by age and time groups for locally confined colorectal cancer

Regional

Survival is unchanged over the 30-year period of this study. Just about half of the patients diagnosed in this stage will ultimately succumb to their disease (Fig. 6.3), the other half are probably cured by surgery. Neither radiotherapy nor chemotherapy is of particular use in this stage. Death from the disease after 5 years is a factor, and late recurrence is not unusual.
Obviously there is a great need to develop means of systemic therapy, particularly as adjuvant to potentially curative surgery, in this stage of the disease.

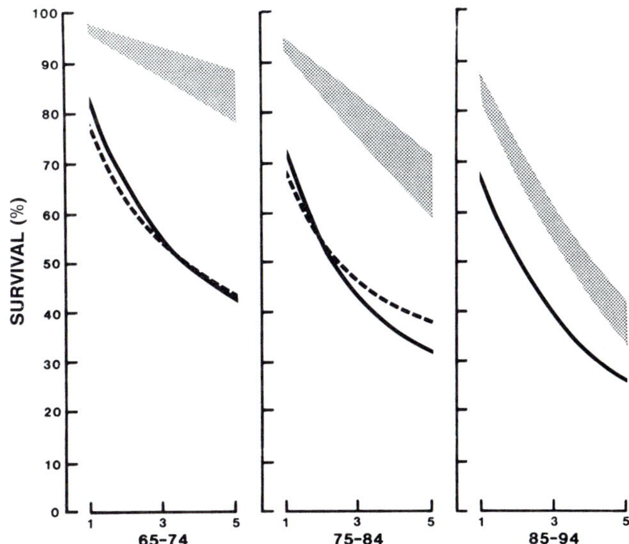

Fig. 6.3. Years survival by age and time groups for regionally spread colorectal cancer

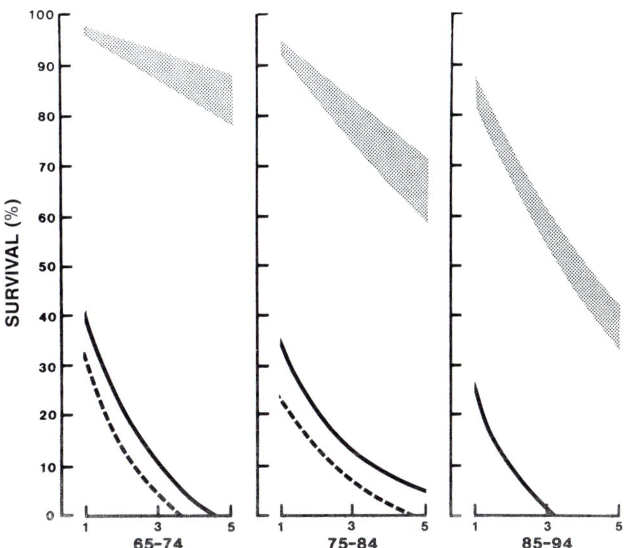

Fig. 6.4. Years survival by age and time groups for distantly spread colorectal cancer

Distant

Just about 15% of all cases of colorectal cancer are diagnosed at this stage, with little variation among the three age groups and between the two time periods. Virtually all patients with this stage of disease die of or with the cancer. The modest increases in survival are only apparent and not significant (Fig. 6.4). The apparent survival past 5 years for the 1970–1979 curve of the 75–84 age-group is an artifact; no patient actually lived beyond 5 years in this group. Until systemic therapy becomes efficacious in this stage of the disease there will be little change in the survival curves.

References

Castleman B, Krickstein HI (1962) Do adenomatous polyps of the colon become malignant? N Engl J Med 267: 469–475

Clarke DN, Jones PF, Needham CD (1980) Outcome in colorectal carcinoma: seven-year study of a population. Br Med J 280: 431–435

Gilbertsen VA, Nelms JM (1978) Prevention of invasive canicer of the rectum. Cancer 41: 1137–1139

Li MC, Ross ST (1976) Chemoprophylaxis for patients with colorectal cancer. JAMA 235: 2825–2828

Miller DR, Allbritten FF (1976) Carcinoma of the colon and rectum: a review of the results of surgical treatment in 164 patients. Arch Surg 111: 692–696

Papillon J (1975) Resectable rectal cancers, treatment by curative endocavitary irradiation. JAMA 231: 1385–1387

Rhodes JB, Holmes FF, Clark GM (1977) Colorectal carcinoma decreasing distally and increasing proximally. JAMA 238: 1641–1643

Sherlock P, Lipkin M, Winawer SJ (1980) The prevention of colon cancer. Am J Med 68: 917–931

7 Pancreas

Cancer of the pancreas is the most discouraging of all human cancers. The incidence has increased by a factor of about 3 in America since 1930. Although several factors may be related to the initiation of pancreatic cancer, none can be considered truly causative. These include cigarette smoking, excessive use of alcohol, and, as recently reported, coffee consumption; most strongly linked is decaffeinated coffee (Bowden 1972; Lin and Kessler 1981; MacMahon et al. 1981).

Pancreatic cancer is indeed a disease of old age. A Mayo Clinic study showed 75% of pancreatic cancer patients in Olmsted County to be 60 years of age or older at diagnosis (Maruchi et al. 1979). Figure 7.1 shows a steady increase in incidence of about sevenfold from age 50 to age 85+. There is a male predominance, but it is not great. Painless jaundice is the classic presentation, particularly in the elderly, but pain and weight loss are common. Until recent years diagnosis of pancreatic cancer was very difficult. However, sonography and computerized axial tomography (CAT) scanning now faciliate diagnosis greatly (DiMagno 1979). Therapy is perhaps the most disappointing feature of all. Surgery is rarely, if ever, curative. Radiation and chemotherapy have essentially no effect (Carter 1980; Mallinson et al. 1980). The major preoccupation of the pancreatic cancer therapy literature of recent years is with the operation that gives the best and longest palliation. This issue is by no means resolved, though some sort of biliary tract diversion seems to be appropriate. Attempts at tumor resection are fraught with high postoperative morbidity and mortality and are rarely justified, especially in the elderly.

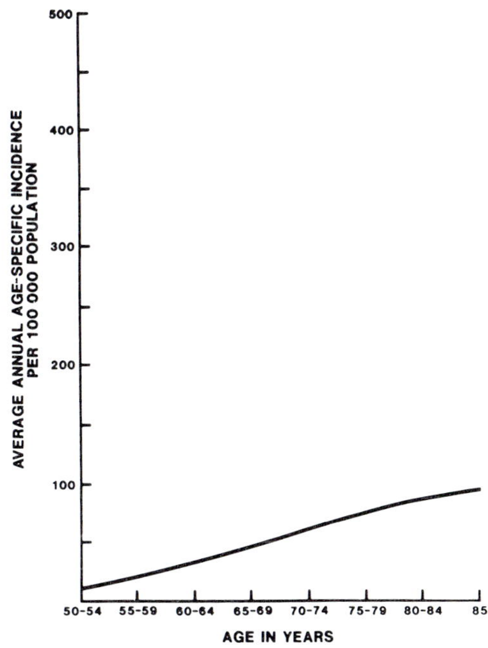

Fig. 7.1. Incidence of pancreatic cancer in USA 1973–1977

Staging pancreatic cancer is an exercise in futility, as survival is the same regardless of stage. Thus, survival data are presented here for all stages combined.

All Stages

Figure 7.2 clearly depicts the first-year mortality of 80%−90% and the incurable nature of this disease. Survival is so poor that age is not a factor for consideration. Interestingly, there is significant improvement in survival at 1 year in the 65−74 age group. This may be due to surgical bypass of biliary tract obstruction. It is difficult to imagine that chemotherapy or radiotherapy have contributed to this small improvement.

This disease usually kills its victim by extension of tumor within the abdomen. It has been amply demonstrated in the past that even the most radical surgical operation rarely separates the patient from all of his cancer, and morbidity and mortality for such procedures are awesome. The rare cure is a Pyrrhic victory if there ever was one. The hope for better management of this disease in the future seems to lie in effective regional therapy that does not cause great morbidity and mortality. Radiotherapy would seem to be the mode of choice if a large enough dose can be delivered to the cancer without irreparably damaging normal structures within the necessarily large treatment fields. There is some early evidence that this area of investigation will prove fruitful in respect of better control and longer survival, though there still may be no real prospects for cure (Borgelt et al. 1978).

The older patient with pancreatic cancer deserves an early attempt to alleviate biliary tract obstruction when it is present and then full attention to palliation. Pain is an almost inevitable consequence of this disease, and its control is usually the most difficult feature of preterminal and terminal care.

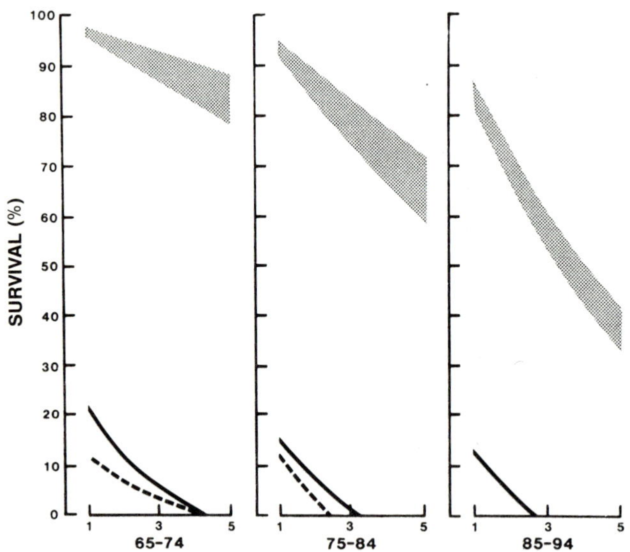

Fig. 7.2. Years survival by age and time groups for pancreatic cancer in all stages

References

Borgelt BB, Dobelbower RR, Strubler KA (1978) Betatron therapy for unresectable pancreatic cancer. Am J Surg 135:76–80

Bowden L (1972) Cancer of the pancreas. CA 22:274–283

Carter DC (1980) Surgery for pancreatic cancer. Br Med J 280:744–746

DiMagno EP (1979) Pancreatic cancer: a continuing diagnostic dilemma. Ann Intern Med 90:847–848

Lin RS, Kessler II (1981) A multifactorial model for pancreatic cancer in man. JAMA 245:147–152

MacMahon B, Yen S, Trichopoulos D, Warren K, Nardi G (1981) Coffee and cancer of the pancreas. N Engl J Med 304:630–633

Mallinson CN, Rake MO, Coking JB, Fox CA, Cwynarski MT, Diffey BL, Jackson GA, Hanley J, Wass VJ (1980) Chemotherapy in pancreatic cancer: results of a controlled prospective randomized multicentre trial. Br Med J 281:1589–1591

Maruchi N, Brian D, Ludwig J, Elveback LR, Kurland LT (1979) Cancer of the pancreas in Olmsted County. Mayo Clin Proc 54:245–249

8 Ovary

Ovarian cancer causes more deaths than any other gynecologic malignancy. Incidence increases somewhat with age above 50, but not greatly. Figure 8.1 shows this clearly. It seems that there are environmental and/or life-style factors that influence this disease, as incidence varies widely around the world.

The average patient could be described as an obese woman in late middle age who had no pregnancies because of infertility (Beral et al. 1978; Cassagrande et al. 1979). This of course implies endogenous hormonal disturbance similar to women with breast cancer. To compound this aspect, it has been shown that there is an increased use of postmenopausal estrogens in women with ovarian cancer as compared with controls (Hoover et al. 1977). This factor alone has considerable relevance for older women.

The capacious female pelvis allows considerable growth of a primary ovarian cancer before increase in abdominal girth or pain alert the patient to its presence. Initial presentation at an advanced stage is all too common. Other than periodic pelvic examination there is no way to screen populations of women for this tumor, which may at any event spread to peritoneal surfaces long before it causes a good-sized mass.

Surgical treatment can be curative, but the majority of ovarian cancers are beyond the chance of surgical cure even at initial diagnosis. Radiation delivered in several different manners has proved to be effective in controlling tumor growth in many instances and is widely used. In contrast to other gynecologic malignancies, chemotherapy has long been known to be useful in controlling metastatic ovarian cancer in a sizable proportion of

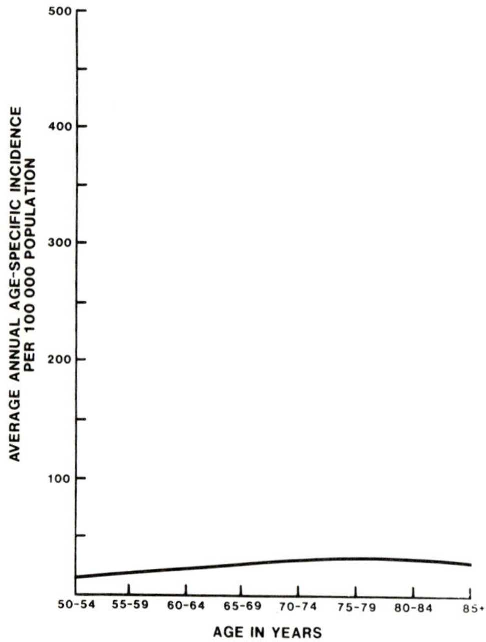

Fig. 8.1. Incidence of ovarian cancer in USA 1973–1977

women with advanced disease. Single drugs, usually an alkylating agent, and lately multi-agent treatment schemes have been surprisingly effective in some reported studies (Tobias and Griffiths 1976; Bagley et al. 1972; Young et al. 1978; Katz et al. 1981).

Local

There are not enough cases to provide comparisons of the two time periods or even to give a reliable survival curve for the 85−94 age-group for the more recent period. Only 20%−25% of ovarian cancers are diagnosed when locally confined. However, when this is the case most women are cured, and in the 75−84 age-group 5-year survival approaches that of the general population (Fig. 8.2). One might conjecture that locally confined ovarian cancer is probably even less a mortality factor in the oldest group of women. Obviously, surgical treatment is the reason for this success, by completely separating the patient from the cancer.

Regional

When the cancer is spread into the pelvis, survival decreases markedly as shown in Fig. 8.3. There are even some deaths from the cancer after 5 years. Unfortunately there are not enough cases to allow comparison between the two time periods or to plot a survival curve at all for the oldest group. This stage accounts for about 25%−30% of all ovarian cancers, and most women die with or of this cancer in this stage. Some women are cured at this stage, but not many.

There are two clear challenges for this stage. The true cure rate, which is probably about 15% overall, might be improved by chemotherapy and/or radiotherapy adjuvant to potentially curative surgery, similar in concept to current management of regionally spread breast cancer.

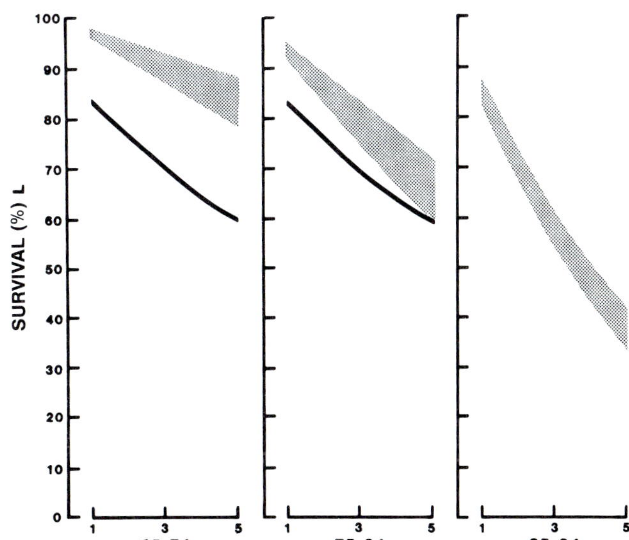

Fig. 8.2. Years survival by age and time groups for locally confined ovarian cancer

The other challenge is improvement in the control of disease not cured. There is reason to believe that radiotherapy and chemotherapy regimens can be improved for patients with residual disease after surgery or recurrent disease later. The good results in widespread disease raise expectations here.

Distant

Just about half of the cases of ovarian cancer have reached this stage by the time of diagnosis. At present there is no hope for cure at this stage, and all women so afflicted will die of or with their disease. Figure 8.4 shows survival to be very poor, but there is

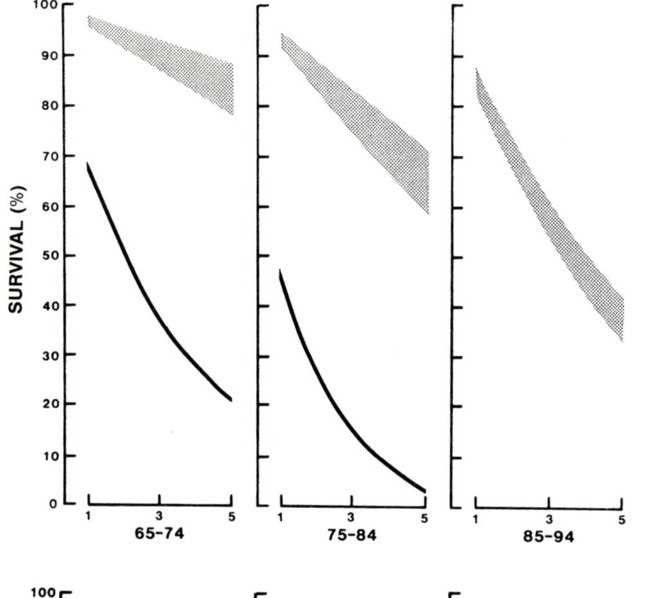

Fig. 8.3. Years survival by age and time groups for regionally spread ovarian cancer

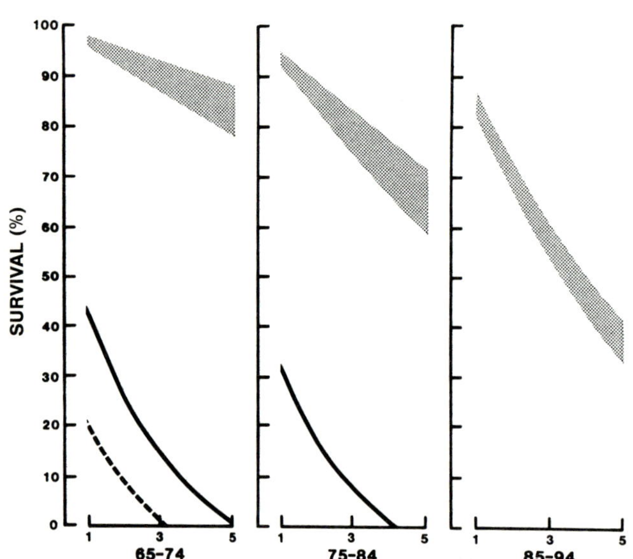

Fig. 8.4. Years survival by age and time groups for distantly spread ovarian cancer

significant improvement at 1 and 2 years in the 65−74 age-group, and apparent increase beyond this. Unfortunately there is not a sufficient number of cases for comparison in the two older age-groups, but there is reason to believe that survival is increased there, too.

Of all visceral carcinomas, that of ovarian origin has proved more responsive to radiation and chemotherapy than most other common types. As systemic disease requires systemic treatment, it might be hoped that treatment regimens will continue to be improved. In that older women are also likely to benefit from chemotherapy in this stage of disease, as apparent from Fig. 8.4, it might be further hoped that drug regimens of minimal or at least acceptable toxicity will be developed. When life expectancy is short − considerably less than 1 year at this stage − chemotherapy is best adapted for outpatient administration, and toxicity should not be great unless a really remarkable regimen is developed.

References

Bagley CM, Young RC, Canellos GP, DeVita VT (1972) Treatment of ovarian carcinoma: possibilities for progress. N Engl J Med 287:856−862

Beral V, Fraser P, Chilvers C (1978) Does pregnancy protect against ovarian cancer? Lancet 1:1083−1086

Casagrande JT, Louie EW, Pike MC, Roy S, Ross RK, Henderson BE (1979) Incessant ovulation and ovarian cancer. Lancet 2:170−172

Hoover R, Gray LA, Fraumeni JF (1977) Stilboestrol (diethylstilbestrol) and the risk of ovarian cancer. Lancet 2:533−534

Katz ME, Schwartz PE, Kapp DS, Luikert S (1981) Epithelial carcinoma of the ovary: current strategies. Ann Intern Med 95:98−111

Tobias JS, Griffiths CT (1976) Management of ovarian carcinoma. N Engl J Med 294:818−823, 877−882

Young RC, Chabner VA, Hubbard SP, Fisher RI, Bender RA, Anderson T, Simon RM, Canellos GP, DeVita VT (1978) Advanced ovarian carcinoma: a prospective clinical trial of melphalan (L-PAM) versus combination chemotherapy. N Engl J Med 299:1261−1266

9 Uterine Corpus

Most cancers of the endometrial lining of the uterus occur after menopause. Indeed, postmenopausal vaginal bleeding is the most common presenting symptom, and enlargement of the uterus is the most common sign at physical examination in this disease. As Fig. 9.1 shows, the peak age of incidence is the late fifties and early sixties. There is a substantial, though declining, incidence into the eighties, however. During the past 10 years or so the incidence has markedly increased, to the greatest degree in the 50–70-year age part of the curve, creating a strange biomodal distribution. In cancer incidence this usually indicates two separate inciting factors, perhaps in this instance reflecting disease from increased use of estrogens immediately after menopause. Because this cancer is eminently treatable with excellent survival prospects in early stages, it is to the great benefit of the patient to detect it early. The only screening mechanism is periodic pelvic examination. The most efficient diagnostic strategy is careful investigation of any patient with postmenopausal bleeding.

During the past decade there have been many papers in the medical literature reporting increased incidence of endometrial cancer related to both premenopausal and post-menopausal estrogen use. Certainly, postmenopausal estrogen use is a very important subject when one thinks specifically of the health and well-being of older women. Weiss et al. (1976) pointed out the increase in incidence of endometrial carcinoma in eight areas of the United States during the 1970s. A number of studies were published over a period of several years, and were vigorously criticized or defended in editorials, and some semblence

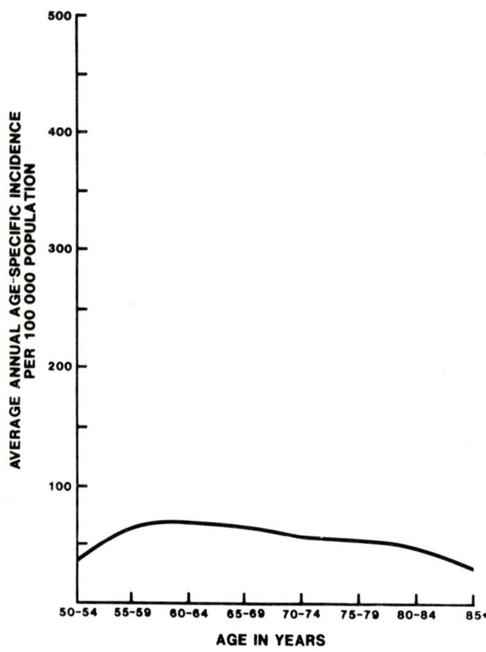

Fig. 9.1. Incidence of uterine corpus cancer in USA 1973–1977

of truth may finally have emerged (Greenwald et al. 1977; Weiss et al. 1979; Shapiro et al. 1980; Weiss-1978; Jick et al. 1979; Hulka et al. 1980). Continuous estrogen stimulation of the postmenopausal endometrium probably does promote the development of endometrial cancer in some women with dose, duration, and formulation of the estrogen all being of importance. The cancer thus promoted is usually fairly well differentiated, not particularly aggressive, and diagnosed at an early stage. Therefore, the mortality for endometrial cancer is not expected to rise in America.

Succinctly stated, treatment is very effective in this disease. Surgery and radiotherapy, singly or in combination, are usually curative in locally confined disease. Nearly 50% of treatment failures are local, so one can make a very good case for hysterectomy whether or not radiation therapy is used. For advanced and recurrent disease chemotherapy has proved of little use.

Local

Just about 75% of all endometrial cancer is presently diagnosed while confined to the uterus, as opposed to about 50% in the 1950—1969 period. This probably reflects earlier attention to postmenopausal vaginal bleeding and could also represent the increased incidence of this cancer in its most differentiated, and thus, least dangerous state, perhaps as the consequence of increased use of estrogens.

Figure 9.2 shows the minimal increase in mortality exacted by this cancer at the local stage in the three age-groups. Also clear is the apparent but not significant increase in survival during the 30-year period of this study. In fact, survival is now so good that it would take a very large number of patients to demonstrate a significant further improvement, presuming that improvement of survival for cancer patients could not be made better than the population at large. At least for the 65—74 age-group one can determine an actual cure rate by use of the 1950—1969 data; it is just about 80%.

The one disquieting feature of this disease is that the percentage of women who die with or of their disease increases with age. Thus, using the 1970—1979 data, the percentages are:

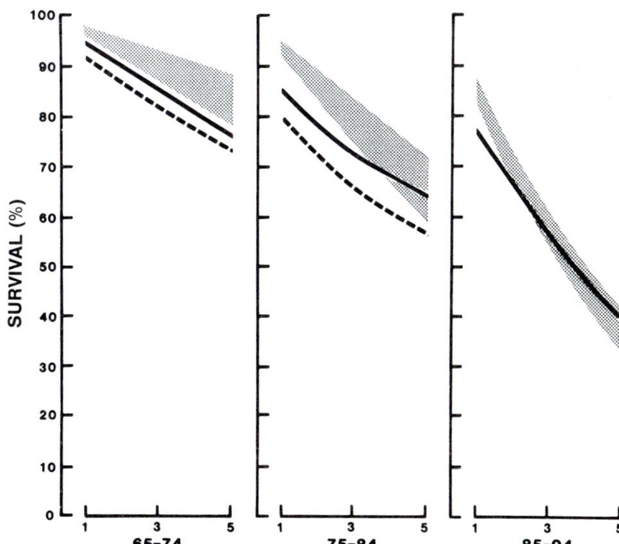

Fig. 9.2. Years survival by age and time groups for locally confined uterine corpus cancer

65−74, 12.4%; 78−84, 16.8%; and 85−94, 34.4%. This might suggest that older women have a more aggressive kind of endometrial cancer than younger women.
When treatment is especially effective, as at this stage of the disease, there is great merit in studying the relatively small number of treatment failures to learn how to modify and improve initial therapy, fine tuning, as it were. The paper of Yoonessi et al. (1979) is a good example of this sort of exercise, and similar studies should be done in the future.

Regional

Spread of this cancer out of the uterus and into the pelvis considerably reduces survival and life expectancy as shown in Fig. 9.3. The absolute cure rate of the youngest group falls to

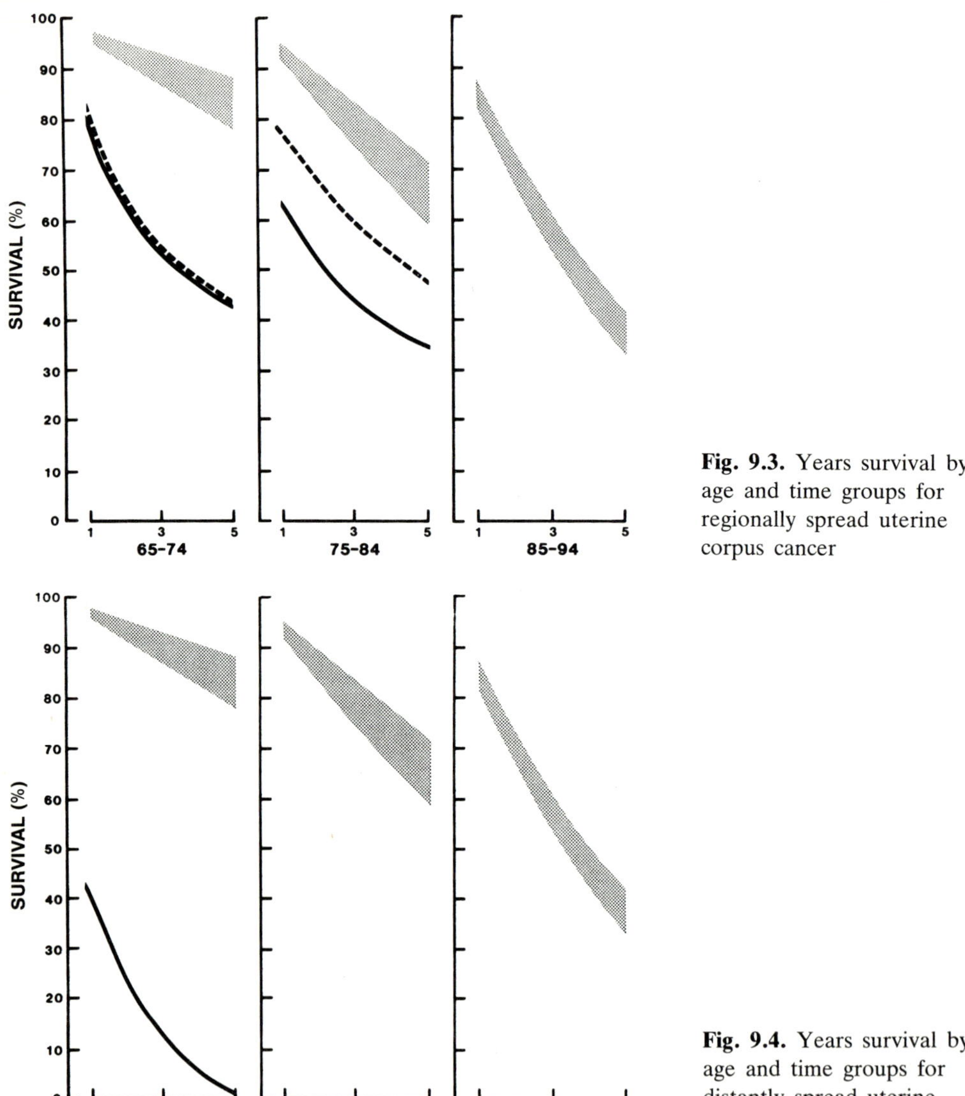

Fig. **9.3.** Years survival by age and time groups for regionally spread uterine corpus cancer

Fig. **9.4.** Years survival by age and time groups for distantly spread uterine corpus cancer

about 50%, and late recurrence of disease becomes a factor to consider. In spite of the fact that survival appeared better among the group of 75−84-year-olds in the 1950−1979 period, there is no significant difference. Treatment by radiotherapy at this stage has been relatively unchanged for many years, as evidenced by the essentially consistent results.

When endometrial cancer progresses to this stage, cure can still be expected. The challenge seems to be careful analysis of treatment failures to provide data for initial treatment modification, though it may be that the limits of effectiveness of radiotherapy have been reached. Unfortunately, chemotherapy and hormonal therapy have been of little or no use in endometrial cancer, so adjuvant treatment schemes are hardly appropriate at the present time.

Distant

This stage of disease is not common, as the single survival curve shows in Fig. 9.4. There is some increase of this stage as a percentage of the whole with increasing age, but it does not exceed 10% even in the 85−94 age-group. It is likely that endometrial cancer diagnosed at this stage is essentially a different disease from the locally confined type. Surely the undifferentiated and aggressive nature of the disease in this stage is obvious.

Systemic disease needs systemic treatment. As mentioned previously, neither hormonal therapy nor chemotherapy appears to alter the course of this cancer. Essentially, all women diagnosed at this stage died of or with their disease. The challenge is clearly to develop multidrug treatment regimens that will not compromise the few remaining months of life by prolonged hospitalization or severe toxicity.

References

Greenwald P, Nasca PC, Caputo TA, Janerick DT (1977) Cancer risks from estrogen intake. NY State J Med 77: 1069−1074

Hulka BS, Kaufman DG, Fowler WC, Grimson RC, Greenberg BG (1980) Predominance of early endometrial cancers after long-term estrogen use. JAMA 244: 2419−2422

Jick H, Watkins RN, Hunter JR, Dinan BJ, Madsen S, Rothman KJ, Walker AM (1979) Replacement estrogens and endometrial cancer. N Engl J Med 300: 218−222

Shapiro S, Kaufman DW, Slone D, Rosenberg L, Miettinen OS, Stolley PD, Rosenshein NB, Watring WG, Leavitt T, Knapp RC (1980) Recent and past use of conjugated estrogens in relation to adenocarcinoma of the endometrium. N Engl J Med 303: 485−488

Weiss NS (1978) Noncontraceptive estrogens and abnormalities of endometrial proliferation. Ann Intern Med 88: 410−412

Weiss NS, Szekely DR, Austin DF (1976) Increasing incidence of endometrial cancer in the United States. N Engl J Med 294: 1259−1262

Weiss NS, Szekely DR, English DR, Schweid AI (1979) Endometrial cancer in relation to patterns of menopausal estrogen use. JAMA 242: 261−264

Yoonessi M, Anderson DG, Morley GW (1979) Endometrial carcinoma: causes of death and sites of treatment failure. Cancer 43: 1944−1950

Cancer of the uterine cervix has long been regarded as a disease of middle-aged women. In recent years there has been great concern about the increasing incidence in young women as well (Mould and Williams 1980). The preoccupation with cervical cancer in young women stems at least in part from the hypothesis that a sexually transmitted infectious agent may cause this cancer, and in part from the great increase in stage 0 − in situ − disease in young women (Beral 1974). In fact, as Fig. 10.1 clearly depicts, the age-specific incidence is nearly constant from middle age through extreme old age for invasive disease.

Invasive cervical cancer, i.e., local and beyond, is totally preventable (Gellman 1976; Macdonald et al. 1973). The Papanicolaou smear (Pap test) has proved to be the most effective cancer screening test devised. Regularly performed on adult females it should reliably detect virtually all stage 0 cervical cancer. Of course, it will detect invasive cancer, too. When asked, most gynecologists will admit that they see relatively few older women as a percentage of their entire practice. Apparently, and understandably, women see gynecologists much less frequently after menopause than before. Accordingly they have fewer Papanicolaou smears. Statistics show that when older women are found to have cervical cancer it is more likely to be invasive than in situ (Siegler 1969). Unfortunately, perhaps, screening for cervical cancer is being attacked as too expensive for the female population at large and strategies are being devised that reduce the number of Pap smears

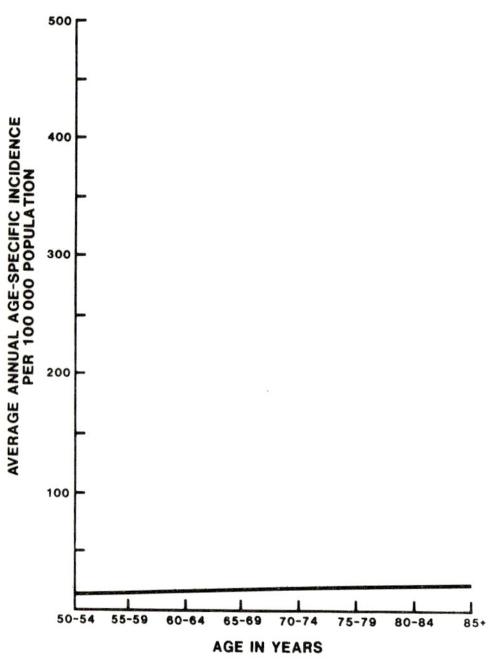

Fig. 10.1. Incidence of uterine cervix cancer in USA 1973−1977 (excludes carcinoma in situ)

that a woman might have in her lifetime (Schweitzer and Luce 1979). Women after menopause get particularly short shrift in these schemes because they have less stage 0 cervical cancer than their younger sisters.

Treatment of invasive cervical cancer is effective at early stages (0 and I) and disappointing at later stages (II and III). Essentially, all women with stage 0 disease are cured, regardless of age. Radiation is the mainstay of treatment for stage I and stage II cancer of the cervix. Stage III cervical cancer is rarely responsive to treatment. Cervical cancer at any stage is basically totally resistant to chemotherapy of any kind.

Several studies seem to indicate that survival in this disease is less a function of age than of the disease itself. Response to standard therapy is as good in elderly as in younger women (Lewis 1966).

Local

Though data for in situ cervical cancer are not included here, it can be summarily stated that survival for women with this disease of any age, including the age-groups of this study, does not vary much from that of the age-matched female population in general.

Figure 10.2 shows the favorable survival when the disease is still locally confined at diagnosis. There is no improvement in the more recent time period but this is not surprising, as treatment techniques have changed little in the past few decades. When not cured, cervical cancer becomes a chronic disease for some women. Usually 5-year survival means cure, but not always. Considerable attention has been devoted to manangement of disease recurring after earlier therapy that was hoped to be curative.

There are special problems in treating older women with cervical cancer because of vaginal and uterine atrophy (Badib et al. 1970). However, as Fig. 10.2 shows, treatment results are really very good, at least in respect of survival.

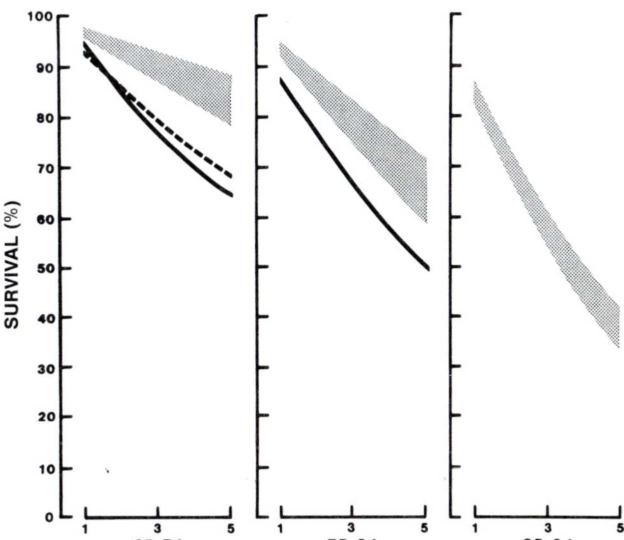

Fig. 10.2. Years survival by age and time groups for locally confined cervical cancer

Regional

Figure 10.3 shows apparent increase in survival for both the 65–74 and the 75–84 age-groups, but in neither instance is this increase significant. There is excessive mortality beyond 5 years for the four curves presented, reflecting both disease persistence and late recurrence.

Of course the great challenge of cervical cancer at any age is detection in the in situ stage and virtual elimination of mortality from this disease. In this day and age there really is no excuse for death from this disease.

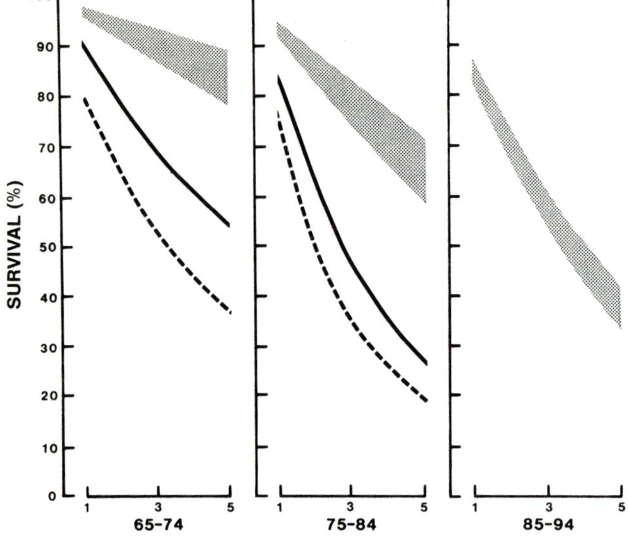

Fig. 10.3. Years survival by age and time groups for regionally spread cervical cancer

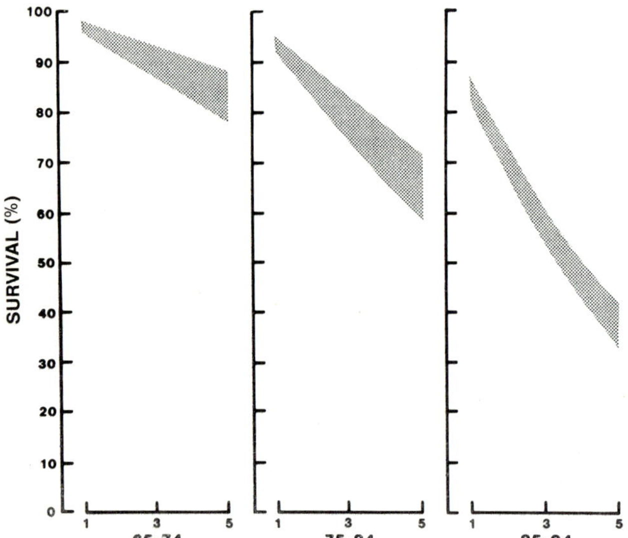

Fig. 10.4. Years survival by age and time groups for distantly spread cervical cancer

Distant

There is not a sufficient number of cases for plotting survival curves for any of the three age groups (Fig. 10.4). Perhaps this is a good omen, because distantly spread cervical cancer is essentially an untreatable disease. For all intents and purposes chemotherapy is without effect.

References

Badib AO, Kurohana SS, Webster JH (1970) Radiotherapy of carcinoma of the cervix in the aged. Geriatrics 25: 108−112

Beral V (1974) Cancer of the cervix: a sexually transmitted infection? Lancet 1: 1037−1040

Gellman DD (1976) Epidemiology and natural history of carcinoma of the cervix. Can Med Assoc J 114: 1003−1012

Lewis DR (1966) Management of cervical carcinoma in the elderly patient. J Arkansas Med Soc 63: 109−111

Macdonald EJ, Morgan JR, Hart MS, Jeserun HM (1973) Incidence and curability of cancer of the uterine cervix in El Paso County 1944−1967. J Am Med Wom Assoc 28: 19−30

Mould RF, Williams RJ (1980) Age distribution of cancer of the cervix uteri. Br Med J 280: 366

Schweitzer SO, Luce BR (1979) A cost-effective approach to cervical cancer detection. National Center for Health Services Research, US Public Health Service, Bethesda (DHEW Publication No(PHS) 79-3237)

Siegler EE (1969) Cervical carcinoma in the aged. Am J Obstet Gynecol 103: 1093−1097

11 Kidney

In the adult, cancer of the kidney almost always occurs as the histologic entity known as hypernephroma or renal cell carcinoma. More common in men than women, by a ratio of 2 : 1, the incidence rises slowly and steadily from ages 50–54 to 80–84, increasing threefold from 11.1 to 34.9 per 100,000 per year as shown in Fig. 11.1.

There are few clues to the cause(s) of these tumors. There seems to be a strong familial tendency and an association with several hereditary syndromes. A recent study by Cohen et al. (1979) even describes association with a chromosomal translocation. However, it would seem that most renal cancers arise sporadically and have no familial background. There is a weak association with smoking, and with residence in an urban as opposed to a rural environment (Wynder et al. 1974; Kantor et al. 1976).

For many years it was thought that most hypernephromas presented with the triad of flank pain, gross blood in the urine, and an abdominal mass. However, it is now known that this presentation is not really very common, particularly among the elderly. Actually a great variety of metabolic abnormalities may herald this tumor, including fever, anemia, erythrocytosis, hypercalcemia, altered liver function tests, and even cardiomegaly (Murphy and Schirmer 1963; Cronin et al. 1976; Pickens 1973; Hajdu et al. 1970).

The growth of hypernephroma is often quite erratic and unpredictable. Even spontaneous regression of metastases has been well documented after removal of the primary tumor. Garfield and Kennedy (1972) reviewed this remarkable phenomenon in 1972 and noted

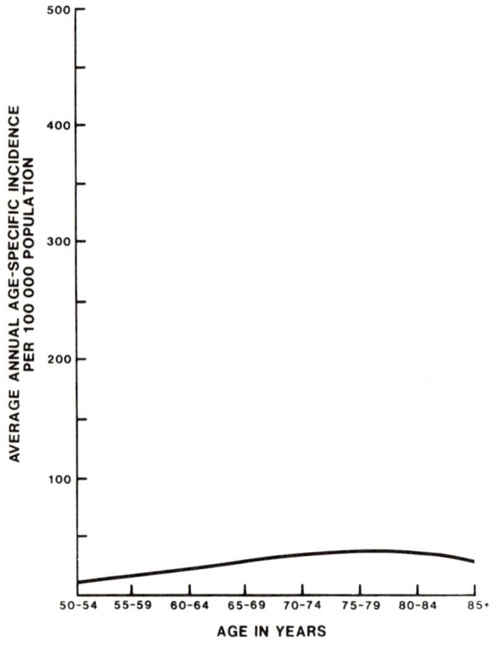

Fig. 11.1. Incidence of kidney cancer in USA 1973–1977

that older males with pulmonary metastases made up the majority of this fortunate group of patients.

Surgery offers the only real hope of cure. Radiation therapy has proved useful for palliation, particularly of painful bone metastases. Chemotherapy has not been particularly helpful in this disease.

Local

In the more recent time period of this study nearly twice as many cases were staged as local as compared with the earlier time period. The significance of this is not clear, but the possibility of generally earlier diagnosis seems quite likely. As Fig. 11.2 shows, there were not enough local cases in the early period to provide meaningful survival curves. Though 5-year survival is not tantamount to cure, the number of deaths from or with disease after 5 years at this stage is very small. This is somewhat in contrast to the impression that kidney cancer is often chronic, with late recurrence a common problem. At present surgery is the only instrument of cure, regardless of the patient's age, and the real benefits of radiotherapy and chemotherapy remain to be demonstrated. This is a very interesting contrast to Wilm's tumor, the kidney cancer of children, where the use of chemotherapy, radiation, and surgery in concert has been one of the great triumphs of oncology. Obviously, treatment failures at this stage are the consequence of disease widely spread at diagnosis but not demonstrable by current techniques. Local kidney cancer offers a good model for development of adjuvant treatment programs at all ages.

Regional

Figure 11.3 shows a considerable increase in survival between the two time periods, which is apparent but not significant with the data available, probably because of the relatively small number of cases. Death more than 4 or 5 years after diagnosis is uncommon, and the

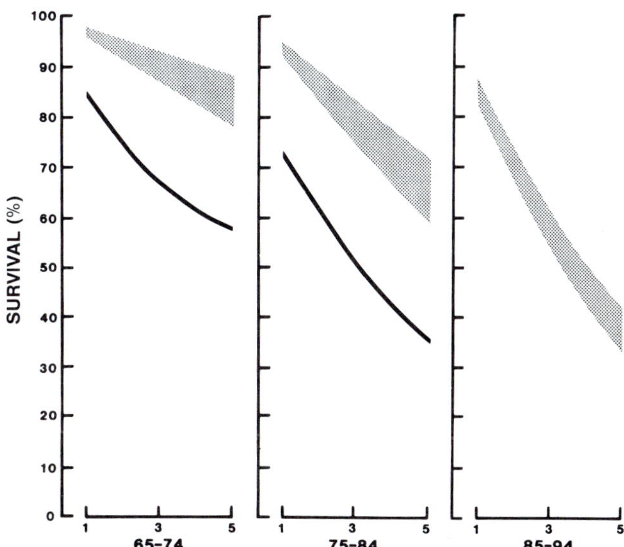

Fig. 11.2. Years survival by age and time groups for locally confined kidney cancer

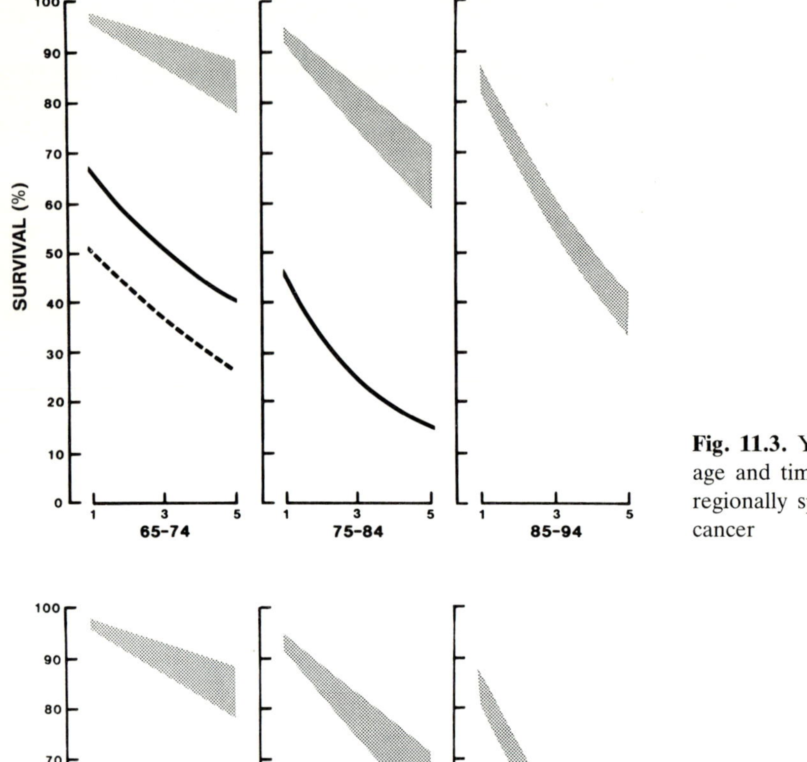

Fig. 11.3. Years survival by age and time groups for regionally spread kidney cancer

Fig. 11.4. Years survival by age and time groups for distantly spread kidney cancer

absolute cure rate at this stage is at least 35%. Obviously, surgery is the sole hope of cure, but radiotherapy does represent a useful adjunct in this stage where the cancer has spread beyond the kidney. Regional kidney cancer also offers a good model for development of adjuvant treatment regimens in the future.

Distant

All patients in this stage of kidney cancer will die with or of their cancer, but a few survive quite a long time, as shown for the 65–74 age-group in Fig. 11.4. There has been no real improvement in survival during the 30 years of this study, which probably reflects the lack of effect of chemotherapy on disease metastatic to bone, lung, and brain.

References

Cohen AJ, Li FP, Berg S, Marchetto OJ, Tsai S, Jacobs SC, Brown RS (1979) Hereditary renal-cell carcinoma associated with a chromosomal translocation. N Engl J Med 301:592–595

Cronin RE, Kaehny WD, Miller PD, Stables DP, Gabow PA, Ostroy PR, Schreier RW (1976) Renal cell carcinoma: unusual systemic manifestations. Medicine 55:291–310

Garfield DH, Kennedy BJ (1972) Regression of metastatic renal cell carcinoma following nephrectomy. Cancer 30:190–196

Hajdu SI, Berg JW, Foote FW (1970) Clinically unrecognized silent renal-cell carcinoma in elderly cancer patients. J Am Geriatr Soc 18:443–449

Kantor ALF, Meigs JW, Heston JF, Flannery JT (1976) Epidemiology of renal cell carcinoma in Connecticut, 1935–1973. J Natl Cancer Inst 57:495–500

Murphy GP, Schirmer HK (1963) Diagnosis and treatment of hypernephroma. Geriatrics 18:354–360

Pickens S (1973) Hypernephroma presenting as cardiomegaly. Br Med J 3:678–679

Wynder EL, Mabuchi K, Whitmore WF (1974) Epidemiology of adenocarcinoma of the kidney. J Natl Cancer Inst 53:1619–1634

Bladder cancer is very much an affliction of older men, though it is less common than prostate cancer. The incidence doubles with every 10 years of age from 50—54 to 80—84, as shown by the increase from 16.5 to 131.2 per 100,000 in Fig. 12.1. Though women get bladder cancer, the male-to-female ratio is about 4 : 1.

Bladder cancer is the quintessential occupational or environmental disease. Rehn (1895) described the relationship of bladder cancer to chemical exposure in the dye industry in Germany in 1895. Studies since have implicated several compounds and it seems likely there are others yet unknown. It takes a mean exposure time of more than 20 years to produce a bladder cancer in this setting, and more than 25% of workers sufficiently exposed will eventually develop this tumor. Beyond this there is, once again, a strong association with cigarette smoking (Cobb and Ansell 1965). This has been known for many years and confirmed over and over again. Most patients with bladder cancer are cigarette smokers, though only a small number have known industrial exposure. In recent years, initially on the basis of animal experiments, saccharin and other artificial sweetening agents have been implicated in the genesis of bladder cancer. The issue is not resolved; there are good retrospective human case-control studies suggesting both cause and no-cause (How et al. 1977; Kessler and Clark 1978).

No one modality of treatment has proved efficacious for invasive bladder cancer. During the past 20 years it has been appreciated that radiation to the bladder followed by total surgical removal is the best therapy for early invasive bladder cancer (DeWeerd and Colby

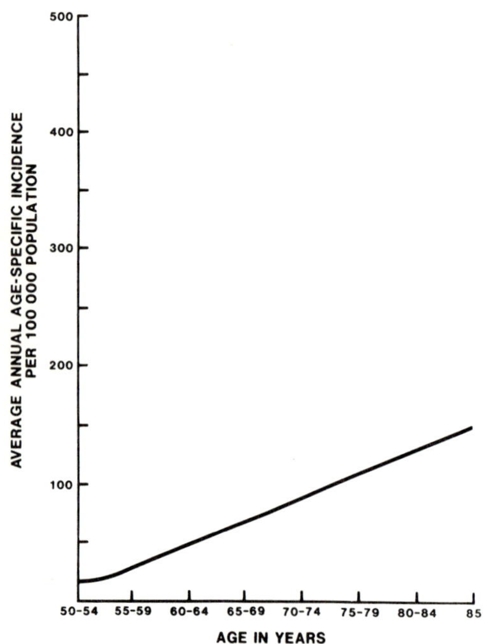

Fig. 12.1. Incidence of bladder cancer in USA 1973—1977

1967). Chemotherapy has been essentially useless in the treatment of advanced or recurrent disease (Caldwell 1974).

Far and away the most common presenting symptom of bladder cancer is hematuria. However, urgency and frequency of urination are also common early in the disease and are often attributed to the prostatism so common in elderly men.

Local

At this stage bladder cancer tends to be a chronic illness; it does not have high early mortality but continues to extract its toll in deaths well beyond 5 years. A much greater percentage of patients were diagnosed at local stage in the 1970s than in the earlier time period in all three age-groups. This could well represent more prompt attention to urologic symptoms in these elderly patients. This is a very salutary change because survival is much better in local than regional disease.

Figure 12.2 shows little improvement in survival between the two time periods. With relatively good survival at this stage it is not surprising that excessive mortality due to this disease is barely detectable in the 85–94 age-group. There is not much room left for improvement of survival; the challenge seems to be improvement of initial therapy and development of better methods of salvage of treatment failures.

Radiotherapy and surgery in combination have become the standard treatment for this stage, but possibly the ideal timing of these two modalities has yet to be realized. Such techniques as intraoperative radiotherapy directly into the bladder are just beginning to be explored. Adjuvant chemotherapy has yet to prove its usefulness.

Regional

Once cancer has spread beyond the bladder the survival rate drops precipitously. As Fig. 12.3 shows, there is high initial mortality and most deaths are with or of the disease.

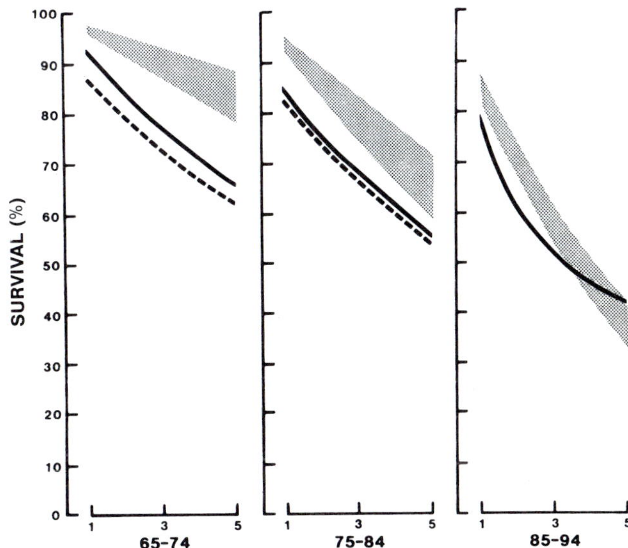

Fig. 12.2. Years survival by age and time groups for locally confined bladder cancer

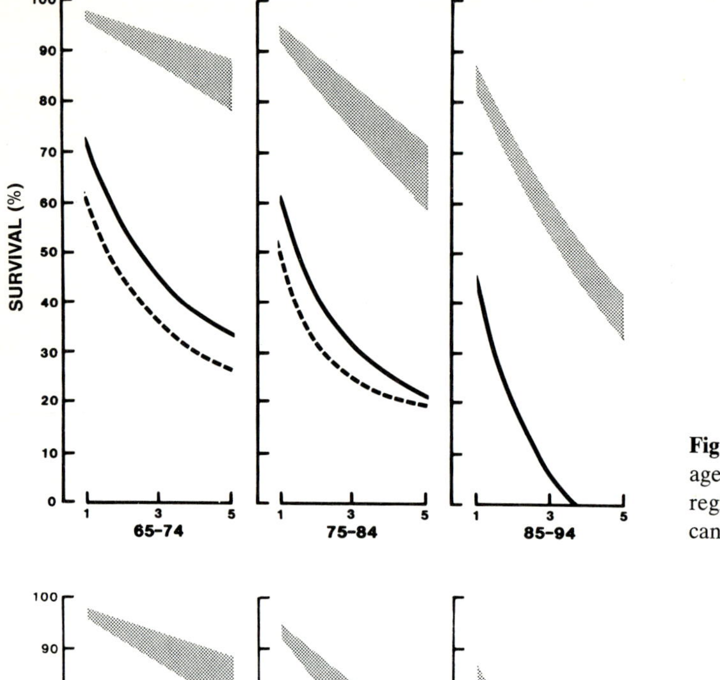

Fig. 12.3. Years survival by age and time groups for regionally spread bladder cancer

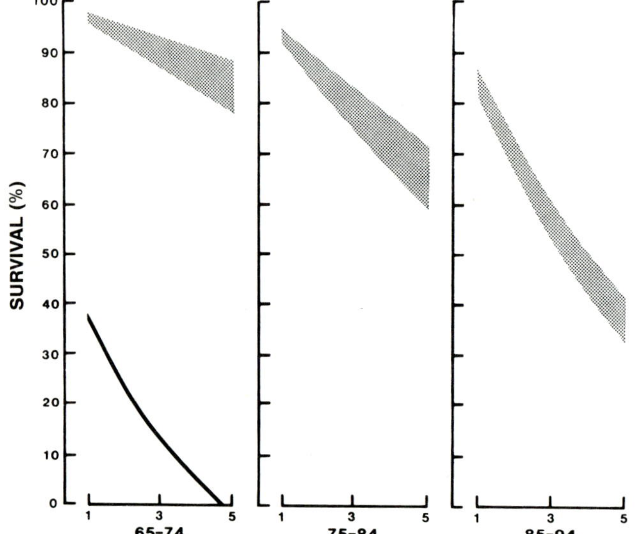

Fig. 12.4. Years survival by age and time groups for distantly spread bladder cancer

However, there is less propensity toward chronicity, and there are few deaths with or of the disease after 5 years. Thus, cure is likely with survival to 5 years, and the absolute cure rate is actually in the neighborhood of 30%. In contrast to the local stage of this disease and to many other regional cancers, there is no mitigation of mortality with advancing age. Virtually all patients in the 85−94 age-group died with or of bladder cancer.

Though survival apparently improved in the 1970s, this is apparent and not significant. Radiotherapy is the mainstay of treatment at this stage and there is obviously considerable room for improvement in survival rates. One can certainly hope that the trend of fewer patients in this stage will continue. Obviously a cheap and effective method for screening for this disease in asymptomatic patients would be of great benefit.

Distant

The number of patients who present with their cancers advanced to this stage is small but, as Fig. 12.4 clearly shows, the outcome for them is poor. Most patients are dead within the first year after diagnosis and all die with or of bladder cancer. Neither surgery nor radiotherapy has anything to offer at this stage other than palliation for the occasional patient. Chemotherapy by single- and multi-agent regimens has proved uniformly disappointing.

References

Caldwell WL (1974) Carcinoma of the urinary bladder. JAMA 229: 1643−1645

Cobb BG, Ansell JS (1965) Cigarette smoking and cancer of the bladder. JAMA 193: 329−332

DeWeerd JH, Colby MY (1967) Bladder carcinoma: combined radiotherapy and surgical treatment. JAMA 199: 109−111

Howe GR, Burch JD, Miller AB, Morrison B, Gordon P, Weldon L, Chambers LW, Fodor G, Winsor GM (1977) Artificial sweeteners and human bladder cancer. Lancet 2: 578−581

Kessler II, Clark JP (1978) Saccharin, cyclamate, and human bladder cancer. JAMA 240: 349−355

Rehn L (1895) Blasengeschwülste bei Fuchsin-Arbeiter. Arch Klin Chir 50: 588−600

13 Lymphomas

The lymphomas are a group of diseases which have in common the fact that the malignant cells look to pathologists as though they derived from cells which normally inhabit lymph nodes. Even when Hodgkin's disease is excluded, as it is in the data presented in this chapter, there is great diversity among the histologic entities which are collectively called lymphoma. During the past two decades many schemes for classifying and relating these entities have been devised, largely based on morphology. It must be admitted that only those specifically interested in lymphomas can keep these classification schemes straight in their minds, that advances in knowledge in this area have been so numerous in recent years that stability in classification will probably not come for some time, and finally that the most usefull classification schemes may be based on factors, other than morphology. As Fig. 13.1 shows, the incidence of lymphoma rises slowly and steadily from middle life into old age. Lymphoma is sufficiently common from childhood through middle age that it cannot be called a disease of the elderly. There is modest male preponderence in incidence. Theories about etiology are numerous, covering viruses, familial factors, chemicals, and induced abnormalities of immunity. Though no human cancer can be said with certainty to be caused by a virus, the lymphomas, particularly Burkitt's lymphoma, are the most likely to have a viral cause (Rigby et al. 1968; Vianna and Polan 1979; Schimpf et al. 1975).

In Hodgkin's disease, as opposed to the lymphomas, meticulous efforts to stage the extent of disease at diagnosis have paid great dividends. In most patients, lymphoma cells are

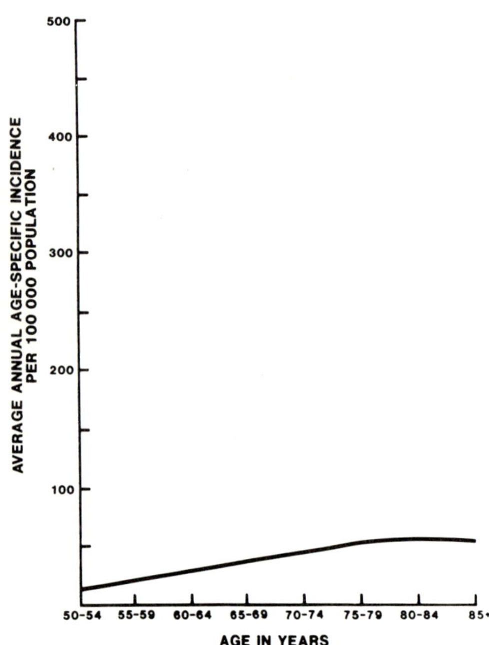

Fig. 13.1. Incidence of lymphoma in USA 1973–1977

probably widespread at the time of diagnosis, though this is often impossible to demonstrate. For this reason radiotherapy has not been the agent of cure that it has been in Hodgkin's disease. Chemotherapy has been effective in controlling the measurable manifestations of the lymphomas, and may often be curative in the most malignant forms, such as histiocytic lymphoma and Burkitt's lymphoma (DeVita et al. 1975; Miller and Jones 1979; Schein et al. 1976).

However, at the other extreme of the spectrum one encounters nodular lymphoma, which may be a very indolent disease. Portlock and Rosenberg (1979) have made a good case for delaying treatment in this fairly common clinical situation. In their controlled series, 4-year actuarial survival of 44 patients for whom treatment was either delayed until clearly necessary or not given at all was 77.3% compared to 83.2% for 112 patients treated at diagnosis ($p = 0.60$).

These data have special relevance fot the elderly, who may not always be good candidates for aggressive chemotherapy. Obviously, great care should be taken in selecting the correct treatment or in delaying treatment for the older patient.

Because stage has less meaning in lymphoma the survival data are presented here in the aggregate, with no attempt to consider the stage at diagnosis. Though it might be useful to separate the various histologic entities and consider the survival experiences separately, this is not really possible because of the many changes in classification according to histology between 1950 and 1979.

All Stages

The slopes of the several survival curves indicate a high mortality in the first year after diagnosis and mortality greater than that for the general population even beyond 5 years. One conclusion is that lymphoma is an acute and rapidly progressive disease for some and a rather chronic disorder for others. Long persistence of disease and late recurrence after good response to initial treatment are common.

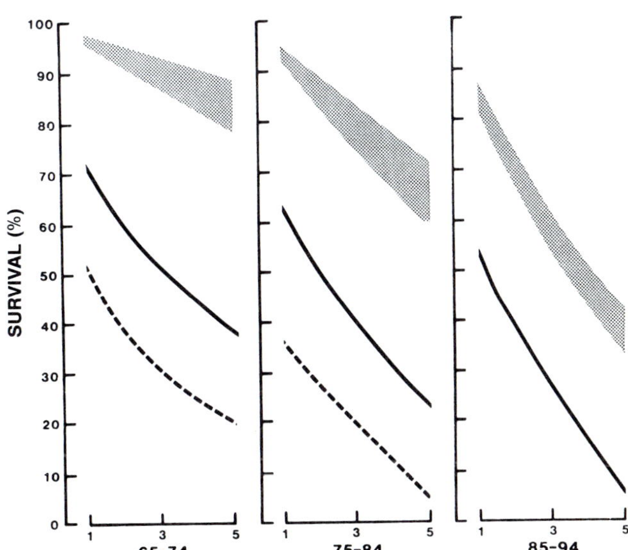

Fig. 13.2. Years survival by age and time groups for all stages of lymphoma

The curves in Fig. 13.2 show a considerable increase in survival percentages over 1–5 years. This increase is statistically significant for all years for both the 65–74 and the 75–84 age groups. There were not enough cases for comparison in the oldest group. There are at least two reasons for this improvement. The first and probably most important is the effect of multi-agent chemotherapy regimens, which gained wide acceptance during the 1970s. They seem to be responsible for better control of systemic manifestations of this disease and are probably curative in a small but definite percentage of the most malignant, that is, histiocytic lymphomas. It is encouraging to note that these effects persist up to the 75–84 age-group.

For elderly patients with lymphoma these data are very important. They provide a clear justification for aggressive treatment of this disease with the expectation of control of manifestations for long periods for most patients, and possible cure of a few, these good effects being obtained regardless of age.

If multi-agent drug treatment regimens can be further improved there is reason to believe that survival may eventually approach that for the general population. In older patients it may ultimately be of little importance to make any distinction between cure and long-term control of this disease.

References

DeVita VT, Canellos GP, Chabner B, Schein P, Hubbard SP, Young RC (1975) Advanced diffuse histiocytic lymphoma, a potentially curable disease. Lancet 1: 248–250

Miller TP, Jones SE (1979) Chemotherapy of localized histiocytic lymphoma. Lancet 1: 358–360

Portlock CS, Rosenberg SA (1979) No initial therapy for stage III and IV non-Hodgkin's lymphomas of favorable histologic types. Ann Intern Med 90: 10–13

Rigby PG, Pratt PT, Rosenlof RC, Lemon HM (1968) Genetic relationships in familial leukemia and lymphoma. Arch Intern Med 121: 67–70

Schein PS, DeVita VT, Hubbard S, Chabner BA, Canellos GP, Berard C, Young RC (1967) Bleomycin, adriamycin, cyclophosphamide, and prednisone (BACOP) combination chemotherapy in the treatment of advanced diffuse histiocytic lymphoma. Ann Intern Med 85: 417–422

Schimpff SC, Schimpff CR, Brager DM, Wiernik PH (1975) Leukaemia and lymphoma patients interlinked by prior social contact. Lancet 1: 124–128

Vianna NJ, Polan A (1979) Lymphomas and occupational benzene exposure. Lancet 2: 1394–1395

14 Multiple Myeloma

This malignancy has fascinated physicians for more than 100 years because it produces easily identified tumor markers, the M protein and the Bence Jones protein. The plasma cell normally resides in the bone marrow. When it becomes malignant it spreads through the red marrow of bones in a manner similar to the leukemias, crowding out normal marrow elements. Unchecked, this leads to anemia, bleeding, and infection. Death occurs from one or more of these problems. The course of illness in plasma cell myeloma is considerably more complicated than in the leukemias because humoral immunity is compromised by insufficient antibody production by normal plasma cells as the number of these cells decreases. The M protein and the Bence Jones protein damage kidney function. However, the hallmark of the disease is bone destruction, either by the malignant cells or mediated through osteoclasts as shown by Mundy et al. (1974). Finally, hypercalcemia and excess urates may cause further problems in this unusual disease. Very little is known of the factor or factors which may incite myeloma, but radiation and excessive stimulation of immunity seem to be possibilities (Matanoski et al. 1975; Isobe and Osserman 1971). Myeloma is slightly more common in men than in women and is very rare before age 50. Incidence climbs steadily from 4.8 per 100,000 per year at ages 50—54 to 30.8 per 100,000 per year at ages 75—79, declining slightly after that as shown in Fig. 14.1. This is, indeed, a disease of the elderly. Diagnosis is often delayed because bone pain in the elderly suggests osteoporosis or metastatic carcinoma to many physicians before it suggests multiple myeloma. Typical plasma cell changes detected on bone marrow aspiration or biopsy permit definitive diagnosis.

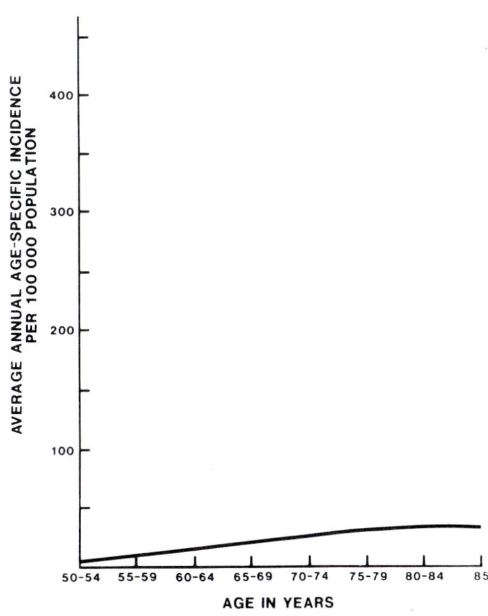

Fig. 14.1. Incidence of multiple myeloma in USA 1973—1977

Occasionally the disease is localized to a single bony area and can then be considered local in extent. However, the vast majority are widespread at diagnosis, though the malignant plasma cells may not be uniformly distributed throughout the red marrow. Thus, marrow obtained from a single site will not always be diagnostic.

A malignant disease of protean manifestations with easily measured markers and a relatively short survival is bound to attract the attention of medical investigators. Plasma cell myeloma has done just that over the past 20 years or so. It has been characterized, categorized, and classified, and innumerable treatment schemes have been tested (Conklin and Alexanian 1975; Midwest Cooperative Chemotherapy Group 1964). No regimen has really proved better than melphalan, an alkylating agent, and prednisone (Brook et al. 1973; Southeastern Cancer Study Group 1975; Hoogstraten 1981).

Median duration of survival after diagnosis has been 24−30 months. In spite of this there are a few patients who seem to do well, regardless of treatment. This entity is often called smouldering multiple myeloma (Kyle and Greipp 1980).

All Stages

No special consideration is given to myelomas of apparently limited extent in this study; rather all stages are analyzed together. Figure 14.2 shows a significant improvement in survival at all years for the 65−74 age-group, and significant improvement at 1 and 2 years for the 75−84 age-group. There were insufficient cases for plotting a 1950−1969 curve for the 85−94 age-group, but survival may well have improved for this age group as well. This improvement is somewhat surprising when one considers the rather gloomy comments from many published drug-trial studies. The shape of the 1970−1979 curve for the 65−74 age-group suggests that median survival is at least 30 months.

It is difficult to imagine how much of this improvement is due to drugs which directly affect the tumor cells − for example melphalan and prednisone − and how much is due to antibiotics, blood transfusions, gamma globulin, and better supportive care. Doubtless all factors are of importance. During the 30 years of this study the survival curve seems to have

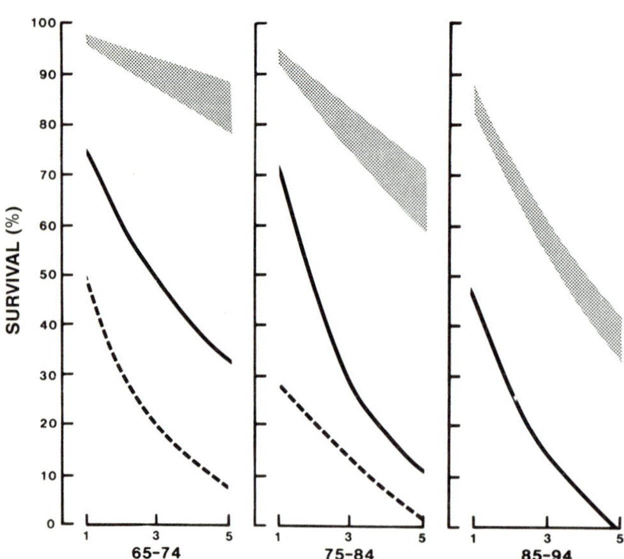

Fig. 14.2. Years survival by age and time groups for all stages of multiple myeloma

moved about one-third of the way up toward expected survival for the age-matched general population. It is likely that we have reached the limits of effectiveness of good supportive care and of the chemotherapeutic agents available, principally alkylating agents like melphalan and cyclophosphamide. Further improvement may only come when new drugs are developed or when innovative methods of reducing malignant plasma cell burden are devised.

Thus, present management of elderly patients with plasma cell myeloma can be conservative. Prevention of infection and of pathologic fractures, or prompt treatment when they occur, may be as important as specific drug therapy. The kidney is the Achilles heel of the myeloma patient, and avoidance of dehydration and sludging of protein in renal tubules is of great importance in management.

References

Brook J, Bateman JR, Gocka EF, Nakamura E, Steinfeld JL (1973) Longterm low dose melphalan treatment of multiple myeloma. Arch Intern Med 131:545–548

Conklin R, Alexanian R (1975) Clinical classification of plasma cell myeloma. Arch Intern Med 135:139–143

Hoogstraten B (1981) Mollites et fragilitas ossium. J Kans Med Soc 82:463–465

Isobe T, Osserman EF (1971) Pathologic conditions associated with plasma cell dyscrasias, a study of 806 cases. Ann NY Acad Sci 190:507–518

Kyle RA, Greipp PR (1980) Smouldering multiple myeloma. N Engl J Med 302:1347–1349

Matanoski GM, Seltser R, Sartwell PE, Diamond EL, Elliott EA (1975) Current mortality rates of radiologists and other physician specialists, specific causes of death. Am J Epidemiol 101:199–210

Midwest Cooperative, Chemotherapy Group (1964) Multiple myeloma, general aspects of diagnosis, course and survival. JAMA 188:741–745

Mundy GR, Raisz LG, Cooper RA, Schechter GP, Salmon SE (1974) Evidence for the secretion of an osteoclast stimulating factor in myeloma. N Engl J Med 291:1041–1046

Southeastern Cancer Study Group (1975) Treatment of myeloma, comparison of melphalan, chlorambucil, and azathioprine. Arch Intern Med 135:157–162

15 Acute Leukemias

Though acute leukemia is not a common cancer of the elderly, it is noteworthy because of its relatively sudden onset, short course, and certain fatal termination. Inspection of Fig. 15.1 shows that incidence slowly rises from the fifties to the eighties, the increase being eightfold between the extremes of ages 50 and 85+. In spite of much conjecture about the possible causes of leukemia, only exposure to significant amounts of radiation and a few chemicals, notably benzene compounds, is known to predispose to this disease, though some familial factors may be of importance (Jablon 1975; Infante et al. 1977). Years spent searching for a viral cause have been largely unrewarded, at least for leukemia in humans (Murphy et al. 1965). A frightening paradox is that acute leukemia is not uncommon in people successfully treated for other cancers (Greenspan and Tung 1974).

A curious feature not obvious in the incidence curve of Fig. 15.1 is that acute leukemia at all ages has a male-to-female ratio greater than one. This is particularly obvious in the elderly, where women outnumber men by a considerable margin in the American population, in the largest published study of acute leukemia in the elderly there were more men than women by a ratio 67 : 36. In adults, especially the elderly, this suggests a greater exposure of men than women to leukemogenic influences of the environment; some focus this on the work place. However, this does not explain the same difference noted in acute lymphoblastic leukemia of young children. Conversely, at all ages females with leukemia live longer than males. Perhaps there are clues in these paradoxes that could be exploited.

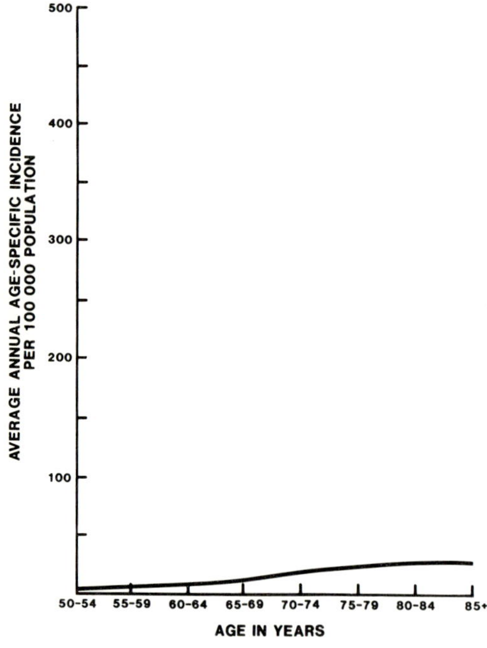

Fig. 15.1. Incidence of acute leukemia in USA 1973–1977

One way to define acute leukemia would be to call it a disease in which a clone of cells develops that do not become senescent. Regardless of the cell line − myelocytic, monocytic, lymphocytic, or another, less common line − the pathophysiology of the disease is the same. Immature cells of a particular clone accumulate in the bone marrow and crowd out normal precursors of red blood cells, white blood cells, and platelets until the patient dies of anemia, infection, or bleeding.

In the past 30 years the treatment of acute leukemia has been, on the one hand, one of the great victories of chemotherapy and, on the other hand, one of the great disappointments. Aggressive multidrug therapy has lengthened mean survival in acute lymphoblastic leukemia of children from 5 months in 1950 to more than 5 years in the 1970s (Pinkel 1971). Indeed, it is believed that some children have been cured of this awful illness. By contrast, the response of the elderly has been very disappointing. Mean and median survivals are little changed in the same 30-year period (Holmes et al. 1979). Death from treatment may be as common as death from the acute leukemia in elderly patients. Even in carefully conducted drug trials it is difficult to determine who died from the disease and who died from the treatment, because the modes of death are the same − bleeding and/or infection. A few elderly people have had excellent response to chemotherapy, with remissions of months or even years, but the question must always be asked at what cost to those who did not respond to treament and who may even have had their lives shortened by it.

There is no disease entity where the ethical issues of active treatment versus no active treatment or versus conservative treatment in the elderly patient are more acutely focused than in acute leukemia. Many have studied this dilemma, but resolution remains to be achieved. As there is no practical staging of this diseasse, all patients are considered stage III or widespread at diagnosis.

All Stages

It is very difficult to find encouragement when considering acute leukemia in the elderly. Figure 15.2 shows an apparent small increase in survival, but it is far from being significant.

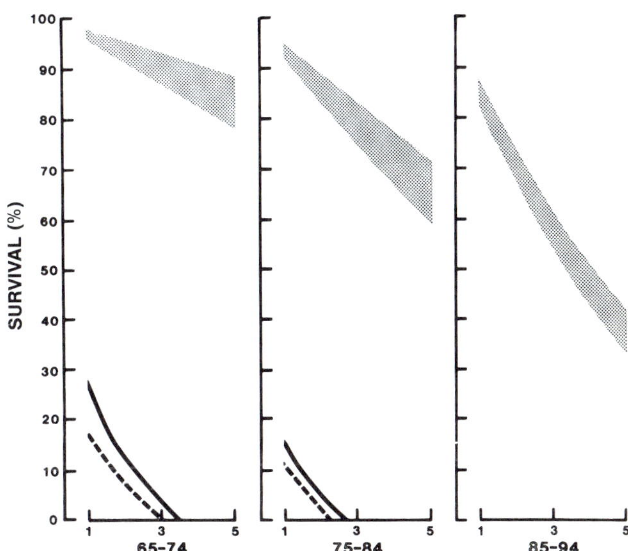

Fig. 15.2. Years survival by age and time groups for acute leukemias at all stages

Both mean and median survival are measured in months. All patients die with or of their disease, the vast majority being in the latter category.

With respect to acute leukemia in the elderly, the challenge is to make the treatment regimens so successful in children and younger adults work in older people as well. Obviously, considerable attention must be paid to histology, which has proved of great importance in treatment response. Even in the elderly, acute lymphocytic leukemia responds more favorably to multi-agent therapy than does, for instance, acute myelocytic or "blast crisis" acute leukemia. However, in the final analysis it is not clear whether the elderly can tolerate the severe toxicity engendered by many multi-agent treatment regimens (Begg et al. 1980).

References

Begg CB, Cohan JL, Ellerton J (1980) Are the elderly predisposed to toxicity from cancer chemotherapy. Cancer Clin Trials 3: 369–374

Greenspan EM, Tung BG (1974) Acute myeloblastic leukemia after cure of ovarian cancer. JAMA 230: 418–420

Holmes FF, Hearne E, Conant M, Garlow W (1979) Survival in the elderly with acute leukemia. J Am Geriatr Soc 27: 241–243

Infante PF, Rinsky RA, Wagoner JK, Young (1977) Leukaemia in benzene workers. Lancet 2: 76–78

Jablon S (1975) Radiation. In: Fraumeni JF (ed) Persons at high risk of cancer, Academic Press, New York, pp 151–165

Murphy WH, Furtado D, Plata E (1965) Possible association between leukemia in children and virus-like agents. JAMA 191: 110–115

Pinkel D (1971) Five-year follow-up of total therapy of childhood lymphocytic leukemia. JAMA 216: 648–652

16 Chronic Lymphocytic Leukemia

Chronic lymphocytic leukemia is a curious disease which has been ignored by medical science for decades. It has excited little interest probably because it tends to be indolent and is found mostly in the elderly. "Found" is a good word because it is almost as often discovered by accident as it is sought because of manifestations of illness. Though the pathophysiology of bone marrow replacement is essentially the same as in the acute leukemias, the course of the disease is measured in years rather than weeks or months.

Figure 16.1 shows its incidence to be 2.6 per 100,000 at ages 50−54 and 35.7 at age 85+, with a straight rise between these two points. The difference is more than 10-fold. At one time in history it was thought that the malignant cell, probably a single clone, was a senescent lymphocyte. Current belief is that the malignant cells usually are B-lymphocytes from a single progenitor cell (Fialkow et al. 1978).

Unfortunately, this change in thought has made little difference in understanding of the disease as there is no clear concept of cause and no agreement on rational therapy. Perhaps the most imaginative kind of treatment is that of Johnson, who has described disease response to low-dose long-duration total body irradiation (Johnson 1970). Lymphocytes generally are easily destroyed by radiation. Chemotherapy is not as efficacious as one might imagine. There is usually involvement of the bone marrow when the disease is diagnosed, and the remaining normal marrow may be more damaged by the drugs than are the malignant lymphocytes. As with acute leukemia, there are twice as many men with this

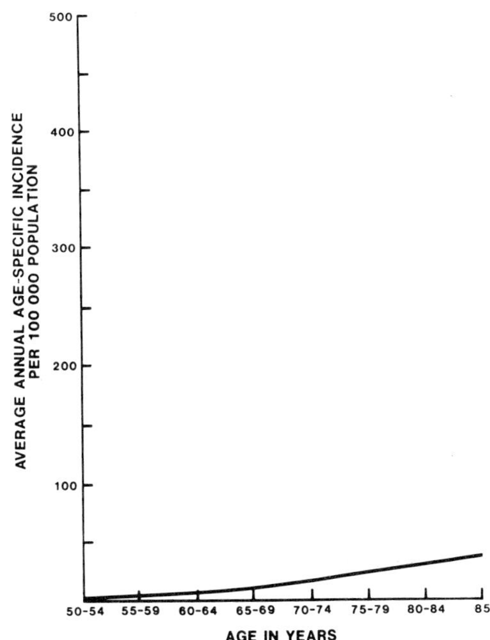

Fig. 16.1. Incidence of chronic lymphocytic leukemia in USA 1973−1977

disease as women, in spite of the fact that older women outnumber older men by quite a wide margin. There is a scheme for classification of this disease devised by Rai et al. (1975), based mainly on extent of disease. However, the patients in this series are presented as one stage.

All Stages

The chronic and indolent character of the disease is clearly portrayed by the survival curves shown in Fig. 16.2. Early mortality is only two to three times that for the general population, but excess mortality persists well beyond 5 years. These are the characteristics of a single chronic disease, in contrast to the lymphomas, for example, and the disease is probably never cured.

Improvement in survival during the 30 years of this study has been minimal and does not even approach significance. This suggests that treatment − almost always chemotherapy − has not altered the course of the disease. Quite a few patients are not treated at all, and a very good case can be made for watchful waiting without employment of chemotherapy or radiotherapy unless compromise of organ function by enlarged lymph nodes or consequences of bone marrow infiltration demand intervention (Holmes and Westphal 1971; Chew and Amare 1980).

Anemia, bleeding, and infection are the consequences of this disease and cause death when not corrected. The past 30 years have seen considerable improvement in management of these problems with blood component therapy and antibiotics. It is even possible that improvement in survival is related to better management of these complications rather than to alteration of the basic course of the disease.

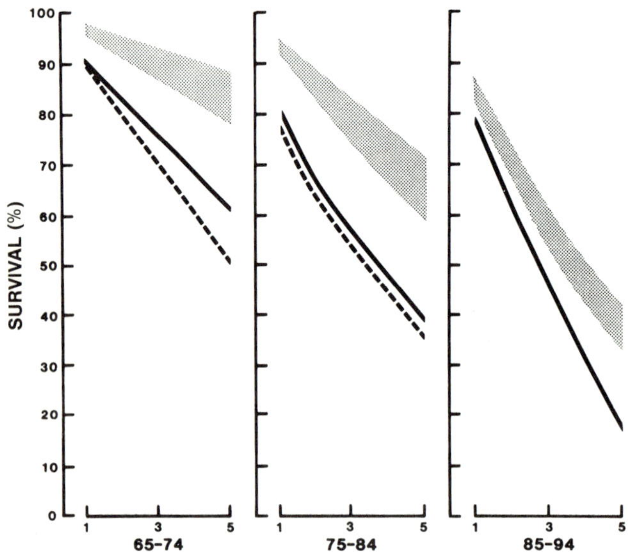

Fig. 16.2. Years survival by age and time groups for chronic lymphocytic leukemia at all stages

References

Chew T, Amare M (1980) Chronic lymphocytic leukemia and related lymphoproliferative disorders. J Kans Med Soc 81: 25−28

Fialkow PJ, Najfeld V, Reddy AL, Singer J, Steinmann L (1978) Chronic lymphocytic leukemia: clonal origin in a committed B-lymphocyte progenitor. Lancet 2: 444−446

Holmes FF, Westphal DM (1971) Survival in treated and untreated chronic lymphocytic leukemia, 1942−1969. Oncology 25: 137−142

Johnson RE (1970) Total body irradiation of chronic lymphocytic leukemia. Cancer 25: 523−530

Rai KR, Sawitsky R, Cronkite EP, Chanana AD, Levy RN, Pasternack BS (1975) Clinical staging of chronic lymphocytic leukemia. Blood 46: 219−234

This variety of leukemia is usually associated with the middle-aged and with young adults. It is not a common disease at any age but the incidence is actually greatest in old age, rising after age 70 and stabilizing at 13−14 per 100,000 per year in the eighties and beyond, as shown in Fig. 17.1. It is equally common in men and women. Fatigue, sweating, and abdominal fullness cause these patients to seek medical attention. Splenomegaly and very high blood granulocyte counts strongly suggest this diagnosis. However, in 1965 Conrad et al. made the point that presentation of this disease in the elderly may be atypical. The relationship of chronic myelocytic leukemia to the other entities in the myeloproliferative syndrome − polycythemia vera, agnogenic myeloid metaplasia, myelofibrosis, acute myelocytic leukemia − is not at all clear.

There is very good cytogenetic and isoenzyme evidence that chronic myelocytic leukemia arises from a single abnormal hematopoeitic stem cell. There is also good evidence that this is an acquired disease. The evidence for radiation exposure as a causative agent is very good; however, because most patients do not have a history of radiation exposure it is likely that there are also other environmental factors which are causative. Considering the fact that incidence increases into the eighties and that the disease is equally common in men and women, it is likely that the environmental agent or agents are ubiquitous and not occupational (Koeffler and Golde 1981).

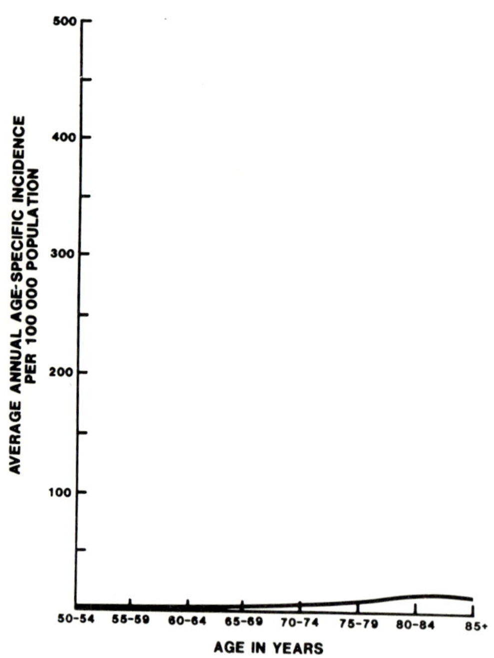

Fig. 17.1. Incidence of chronic myelocytic leukemia in USA 1973−1977

The course of the disease is measured in months to years with termination in "blast crisis," a kind of acute leukemia, virtually inevitable. Single-agent chemotherapy, radioactive phosphorus, and irradiation of the enlarged spleen have been tried with some effect but without changing the course of the disease in the majority of patients. A small number have very long remissions. However, the elderly do less well with this disease than the young. The frontier of therapy for chronic myelocytic leukemia seems to be bone marrow transplantation (Goldman et al. 1981). The benefits of removal of the very large spleens in these patients have not been established, though lengthened and more comfortable survival seems to accrue to some (Spiers et al. 1975; Ihde et al. 1976).

All Stages

There are sufficient cases to compare early and late period survival only for the 65–74 age-group. There is no significant difference between these two curves in Fig. 17.2, but the difference in the slopes of the two is interesting and might suggest that the survival pattern is changing. In view of the general improvement of supportive care for patients with all kinds of malignancies in recent years one might wonder why survival at 1 year is decreased to a considerable, though not significant, extent. We still await the demonstration that a particular mode of therapy in this kind of cancer will alter the course of disease for a meaningful number of patients. The increased survival at 5 years in the late period is of interest.

While many therapies, indeed almost any, will reduce high white blood cell counts in this disease, there is no evidence that this alters the natural course of the disease per se. Therapy that removes the Ph[1] clone of cells certainly appears promising (Fefer et al. 1979). For the elderly patient the best strategy at present seems to be conservative.

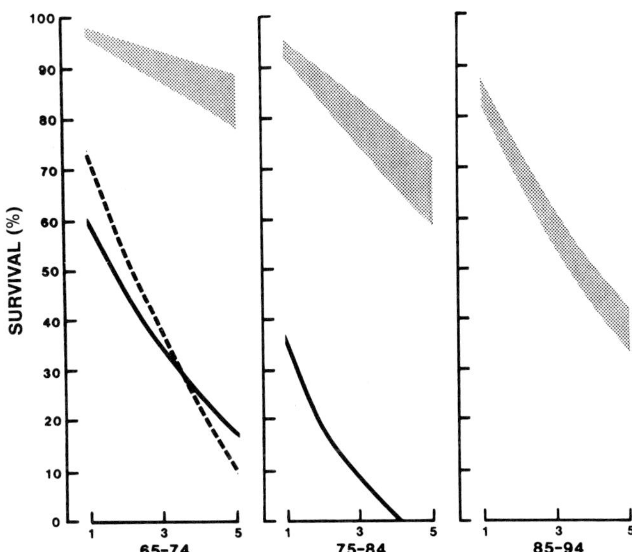

Fig. 17.2. Years survival by age and time groups for chronic myelocytic leukemia at all stages

References

Conrad ME, Rappaport H, Crosby WH (1965) Chronic granulocytic leukemia in the aged. Arch Intern Med 116: 765–775

Fefer A, Cheever MA, Thomas ED, Boyd C, Ramberg R, Glucksberg H, Buckner CD, Storb R (1979) Disappearance of Ph[1]-positive cells in four patients with chronic granulocytic leukemia after chemotherapy, irradiation and marrow transplantation from an identical twin. N Engl J Med 300: 333–337

Goldman JM, Johnson SA, Catovsky D, Wareham NJ, Galton DAG (1981) Autografting for chronic phase of chronic granulocytic leukemia. N Engl J Med 305: 700

Ihde DC, Canellos GP, Schwartz JH, DeVita VT (1976) Splenectomy in the chronic phase of chronic granulocytic leukemia. Ann Intern Med 84: 17–21

Koeffler HP, Gode DW (1981) Chronic myelogenous leukemia – new concepts. N Engl J Med 304: 1201–1209, 1269–1274

Spiers ASD, Baikie AG, Galton DAG, Richards HGH, Wiltshaw E, Goldman JM, Catovsky D, Spencer J, Peto R (1975) Chronic granulocytic leukemia: effect of elective splenectomy on the course of disease. Br Med J 1: 175–179

18 Brain

The incidence of brain tumors is unusual in comparison with other neoplasms because there is a definite decline among the aged, as shown in Fig. 18.1. Brain tumors particularly those in the cerebellum, are relatively common in childhood. Incidence remains fairly constant until the sixties, when there is a steady decline, with the incidence being quite low in the very elderly. The male-to-female ratio is nearly one except for meningiomas, which are about twice as common in women is in men. As the causes of brain tumors are not known, there is no explanation for the unusual incidence patterns. Several good review articles addressing brain tumors in the elderly have been published in the past decade (Tomita and Raimondi 1981; Cooney and Solitare 1972).

Treatment is gratifying and cure possible when a tumor can be completely excised at surgery. When this is not possible, partial excision or radiation therapy are palliative and prolong survival. Chemotherapy has been tried in many modalities in the past two decades, but there have been no conspicuous successes, even with respect to prolonged palliation.

The most discouraging of all brain tumors is the glioblastoma multiforme. It is fast growing, probably never cured, and clearly the most common brain tumor after age 60. Even with maximum effort at palliation by combined surgery, radiation, and chemotherapy, Hochberg et al. (1979) reported median survival of a group of 74 patients to be 11.5 months.

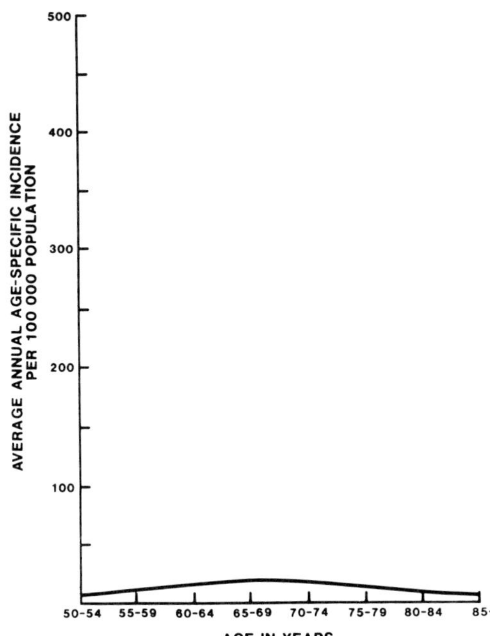

Fig. 18.1. Incidence of brain tumors in USA 1973–1977

Brain tumors are important to older patients because disabling disease of the central nervous system is extremely common in this age group. Actually the most common cancer in the brain is a metastasis or metastases from elsewhere in the body; cancer cells from lung, breast, and kidney commonly spread to the brain. Trauma, often even minor trauma, frequently causes subdural hematoma in the elderly. Confusion, paralysis, and visual difficulties may herald any of these entities. Even if only a few primary brain tumors are curable they need to be identified. In the past, diagnosis of intracranial lesions was difficult; however, CAT scanning and isotope scanning have revolutionized this whole field.

All Stages

Because brain tumors almost never metastasize, all cerebral tumors are considered in this analysis without regard to stage. Meningioma is not included here because it is rare in the elderly, is rarely a cancer, is not a brain tumor per se, and is usually cured by surgery. Metastatic cancers in the brain are also excluded.

Figure 18.2 shows significant improvement in survival at 1 year for the 65–74 age-group and an apparent increase in survival up 5 years. Reasons for this are not clear, but the pattern is consistent with improved control and even raises the possibility that an occasional cure occurs. Increased use of radiotherapy after surgery and liberal use of corticosteroids to control tumor and brain edema have no doubt contributed to improved survival percentages. With regard to survival, age does not seem to be a factor of importance.

Some radical departures seem to be necessary if significant improvements in survival are to be achieved. There are clear limits to how much of the brain can be removed at surgery while preserving the function and personality of an individual. High doses of radiotherapy are delivered to the brain with current techniques, and the normal part of the brain can tolerate these dosages with few immediate ill effects. It is difficult to know how radiotherapy of brain tumors can be improved unless higher energy or different particles

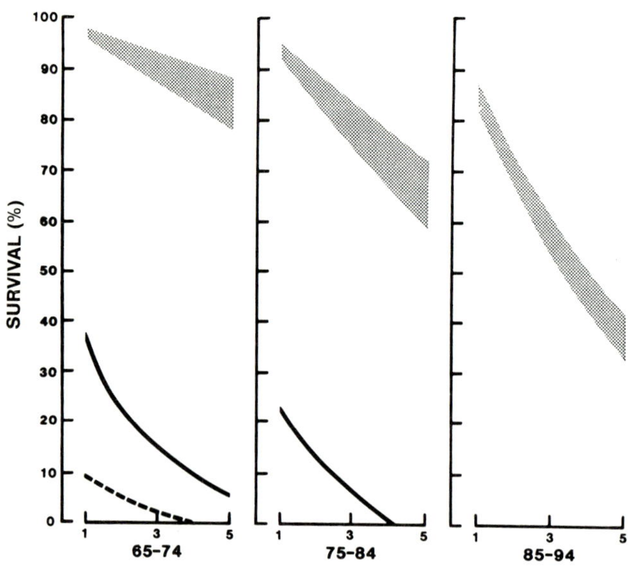

Fig. 18.2. Years survival by age and time groups for brain cancer at all stages

are employed or sources of radiation are implanted in the brain tumor. New and different chemotherapeutic agents are clearly needed since those currently available do not affect brain tumor growth very much.

The elderly patient with a brain tumor deserves at least a biopsy of the tumor to establish the histologic diagnosis to provide data for prognosis, and perhaps to expedite radiation therapy. If radiation therapy is easily available it can usually be given in outpatient treatment with little side effect. The management of the disease thereafter is mostly common sense, with every attempt being made early to keep the patient functioning and active. Pain is not inevitable, and when present it is controllable. Corticosteroids often seem to provide extra months of good life and are beneficial for their tonic and euphoric effects, as well as control of seizures. Increasing neurological and intellectual impairment, coupled with visual compromise, inevitably leads to coma and death. Often a few months of good nursing-home care are necessary.

References

Cooney LM, Solitare GB (1972) Primary intracranial tumors in the elderly. Geriatrics 27:94–104

Hockberg FH, Linggood R, Wolfson L, Baker WH, Kornblith P (1979) Quality and duration of survival in glioblastoma multiforme: combined surgical, radiation and lomustine therapy. JAMA 241:1016–1018

Tomita T, Raimondi AJ (1981) Brain tumors in the elderly. JAMA 246:53–55

19 Primary Site Unknown

Cancer of unknown primary site is a neoplastic bastard, a child without a father. When metastases rather than the primary tumor cause signs or symptoms the diagnosis of cancer is often made from the metastases. More often than not, the search for the primary tumor is successful. Liver metastases usually come from the gastrointestinal tract but may come from very small breast or lung primary tumors. Metastases in neck lymph nodes should be the consequence of an occult primary tumor in the head and neck, but sometimes even primary tumors below the diaphragm metastasize to neck nodes. When the search for the primary source of metastases is unsuccessful, the appellation "primary site unknown" is appropriate. In published series these comprise 0.5%–5% of cancers (Didolkar et al. 1977; Holmes and Fouts 1970).

The best justification for a methodical search for the primary tumor is that its identification may influence treatment, for example the treatment of metastatic breast carcinoma is clearly different than the treatment of metastatic thyroid carcinoma. However, some believe that little more than a perfunctory effort should be made (Stewart et al. 1979; Nystrom et al. 1979). Certainly in the elderly patient with an incurable disease in which survival is short, one can make a good case for placing some limit on the number of tests done to find an elusive primary cancer once the potentially controllable sites – e.g., breast, thyroid, endometrium, and ovary – are eliminated.

As shown in Fig. 19.1, the incidence of this kind of cancer is age related, essentially doubling each decade from age 50 to age 80. Incidence data are for the period 1969–1971

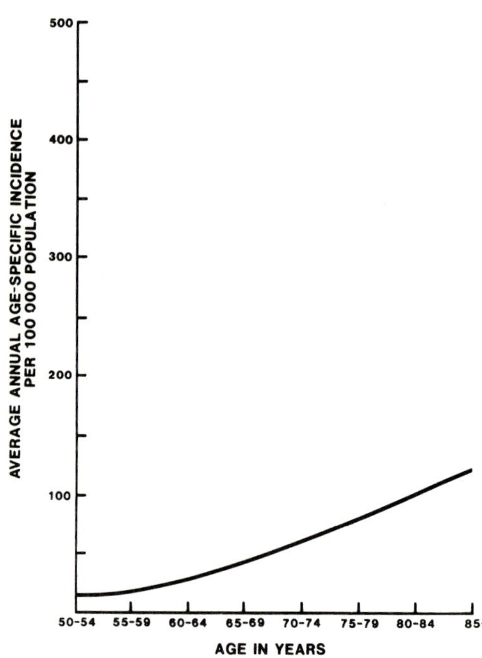

Fig. 19.1. Incidence of cancer with primary site unknown in USA 1969–1971

(Cutler and Young 1975) because they are not available for the period 1973–1977 as in the other chapters. This generally parallels the increasing incidence of cancer with increasing age, but also could reflect the likelihood that the vigor of the search for elusive primary cancers is inversely proportional to age. That this cancer may be an eminently treatable disease has recently been demonstrated by Woods et al. (1980) who found a chemotherapy regimen of doxorubicin and mitomycin-C to be better than a regimen of cyclophosphamide, methotrexate, and 5-fluorouracil.

All Stages

It is inappropriate to stage patients with this disease. None are local, and there is no way to separate those patients who might have regional disease from those who have widespread cancer. Thus, cases are considered together as all stages and might as well be equated with widespread.

In Fig. 19.2 considerable improvement is shown in survival between the late and early time periods in the 65–74 and 75–84 age-groups, with insufficient cases from the early time period to provide a comparison for the 85–94 age-group. This improvement is significant at 1 and 2 years for the 65–74 age-group. Though improved supportive care might be invoked as contributing to this improvement, it probably does not contribute as much as does therapy directed to control of this variety of metastatic cancer. This surely includes both radiotherapy and chemotherapy, and confirms, in a way, the work of Woods et al. (1980), cited previously.

Because this group of patients has a high proportion of undifferentiated and poorly differentiated carcinomas it provides the ideal venue for testing new drug treatment regimens, even in older patients. It seems likely that in past years many of these patients were less than adequately treated, in that they were denied newer regimens because they could not be fit into a specific site protocol. Perhaps additional specific protocols for primary site unknown patients should be devised and tested.

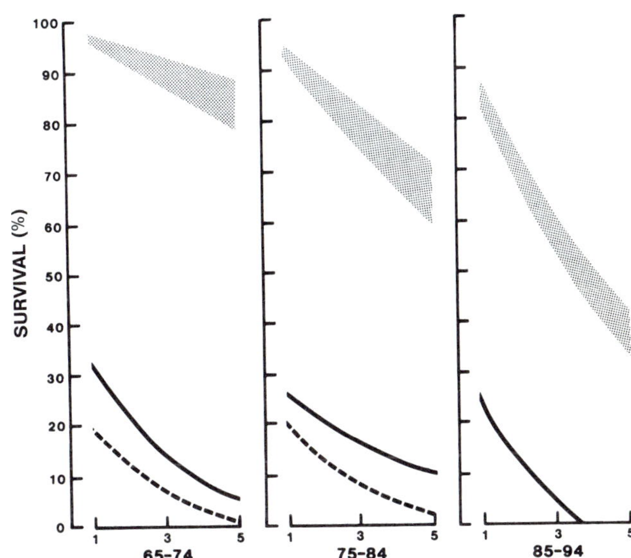

Fig. 19.2. Years survival by age and time groups for primary site unknown cancer at all stages

If histopathology improves, and particularly if the use of various tissue and humoral tumor markers improves in the next few years, there may be fewer patients diagnosed as having primary site unknown cancers. This would certainly benefit frail elderly patients; disease management could then be focused on treatment rather than on finding the elusive primary cancer.

References

Cutler SJ, Young RL (1975) Third national cancer survey: incidence data. National Cancer Institute, United States Public Health Service, Bethesda (DHEW publication no (NIH)75-787)

Didolkar MS, Fanous N, Elias EG, Moore RH (1977) Metastatic carcinomas from occult primary tumors. Ann Surg 186: 625–630

Holmes FF, Fouts TL (1970) Metastatic cancer of unknown primary site. Cancer 26: 816–820

Nystrom JS, Weiner JM, Wolf RM, Bateman JR, Viola MV (1979) Identifying the primary site in metastatic cancer of unknown origin: inadequacy of roentgenographic procedures. JAMA 241: 381–383

Stewart JF, Tattersall MHN, Woods RL, Fox RM (1979) Unknown primary adenocarcinoma: incidence of overinvestigation and natural history. Br Med J 1: 1530–1533

Woods RL, Fox RM, Tattersall MHN, Levi JA, Brodie GN (1980) Metastatic adenocarcinomas of unknown primary site: a randomized study of two combination-chemotherapy regimens. N Engl J Med 303: 87–89

20 Conclusion

The increasing number of elderly people in the American population means that the number of cancer cases will continue to increase unless incidence declines. Though the incidences of stomach and cervical cancers are still declining, they are more than offset by increases in lung and pancreatic cancers. The fastest growing segment of our population is that comprising people 85 and older. The cancer incidence for this group is 2,308 per 100,000 per year; this means that 2.3% of people older than 84 will be diagnosed as having cancer per year. Thus, the data presented in this book are going to be increasingly important as time goes on, and there is a great need to continue these analyses.

The lessons from prostate cancer must not be forgotten. Survival analysis is the final arbiter; only controlled trials prove the efficacy of new treatment methods, and it is not likely that cancer patients can be treated so effectively that they will outlive the population at large. In this regard, breast cancer in elderly women can be seen in interesting contrast to prostate cancer. Survival in locally confined disease just about approximates survival for the age-matched general female population, particularly for those aged 75 to 94. There is ground to gain in regionally spread disease, but not very much. Remarkable progress has been registered in distantly spread disease, probably in large measure as a result of methodical improvement in hormonal and drug therapy by repeated controlled trials during the 30-year span of this study. There is still progress to be made in prevention and management of both early and late recurrence of breast cancer in elderly women.

Though the incidence of lung cancer declines after about age 75, the rates at younger ages in both sexes continue to climb. Lung cancer is curable at any age but only in a small percentage of those diagnosed, and this percentage has not actually changed in 30 years. Perhaps better control should be our immediate goal in dealing with lung cancer. The significant survival improvement at 1 and 2 years in regionally spread disease and lengthened survival in small cell histology may be the heralds of this. Though the normal lung tolerates radiation poorly, it seems likely that improved radiotherapy techniques will facilitate disease control and short-term survival still further. The big question is whether or not effective chemotherapy can be devised to deal with non-small cell histologies. This would greatly facilitate control of noncurable disease and might improve survival rates after potentially curative surgery, as it has in breast cancer.

Considered collectively, gastrointestinal cancers are far and away the major force in cancer morbidity and mortality among the aged in America. It is ironic indeed that as incidence of stomach cancer declines, that of pancreatic cancer inexorably increases, and that incidence of colorectal cancer is stable though there is more right-side colonic cancer and less rectal cancer. We have little understanding of etiologic factors in these disease entities. The irony is compounded by the fact that the efficiency of our treatment efforts remains essentially unchanged and, with the exception of significantly improved 1-year survival in regionally spread stomach cancer in age-group 75–84, is reduced to cure or failure, with control barely a consideration. In this regard it can be stated that, at any age, stomach cancer is rarely cured, pancreatic cancer virtually never, and colorectal cancer in about 50% of cases. Only surgery is effective therapy; chemotherapy and radiotherapy have been of little use. Identifying serum markers of these cancers to make early diagnosis possible, and extending and improving screening for asymptomatic colorectal cancer in the elderly by simple inexpensive detection of occult blood or other substances in stool are appropriate research strategies. Obviously, radically different radiotherapy techniques and chemo-therapeutic agents will be needed to give these forms of treatment credibility in gastrointestinal cancer.

Gynecologic cancer would have a low mortality if every woman, regardless of age, had an annual pelvic examination and Pap smear. The fact that virtually all women now regard postmenopausal vaginal bleeding as abnormal, and that they quickly seek medical advice when it occurs, is probably the reason that endometrial cancer is usually diagnosed at an early stage and usually cured. Unfortunately, cervical and ovarian cancers make their presence known later in the course of the disease, and cure rates are correspondingly lower.

Widespread endometrial and cervical cancers are essentially untreatable diseases by current therapeutic methods, with chemotherapy of little use. When these two diseases are regionally spread at diagnosis, radiotherapy gives relatively good cure rates and excellent control of disease not cured. Though ovarian cancer is not diagnosed at an early stage as often as it should be, surgical cure rates are excellent. Both radiotherapy and chemotherapy make significant contributions to control of regional and widespread disease, and there is every reason to believe that modifications of these modalities will improve disease control in the future.

In contrast to prostate cancer, both kidney and bladder cancer are usually not indolent diseases and are eminently curable when diagnosed at an early stage. Long survival, i.e., greater than 4 years, usually means cure of these two cancers. Kidney cancer cure rates are excellent for locally confined disease and fair for regionally spread disease, while bladder cancer cure rates are even better. Early diagnosis is therefore the key to effective treatment.

Radiotherapy is supplemental to surgery in bladder cancer and useful for palliation in kidney cancer. Chemotherapy is very disappointing in both.

Kidney and bladder cancers occur mainly in men, and it is tempting to compare them with gynecologic cancers in women. In this regard it is unfortunate that screening and early diagnosis in the former are so less well developed than in the latter. Conceptually, exfoliative cytology — the Pap smear — should be nearly as useful in detecting early bladder cancer as it is in detecting early cervical cancer. Unfortunately, this has not been the case. Like the ovary, the kidney lies deep in the body in a place where considerable undetected growth is possible. While many asymptomatic ovarian cancers are detected by physical examination, few kidney cancers are.

Collectively, the hematologic malignancies are a major factor in cancer morbidity and mortality in old age. They range from the most acute to the most indolent of cancers. Some older patients with Hodgkin's disease and histiocytic lymphoma may be curable, but as a general rule it can be stated that hematologic cancers in the elderly are incurable.

One of the surprises of this study is the remarkable improvement in survival in plasma cell myeloma and the lymphomas among aged patients diagnosed in the past 10 years. This improvement is doubtless due to the development of effective chemotherapy well beyond the improvement in survival one might expect from better supportive care. In stark contrast are the leukemias, where no significant survival improvement has been noted in spite of intensive efforts to perfect multiagent chemotherapy and greatly improved supportive care. The contrast within the leukemias is great, too. The acute leukemias have highest mortality and that of chronic lymphocytic leukemia is very low, treatment offering little or nothing in either instance.

For all of the hematologic malignancies future improvement in survival will devolve on better chemotherapy or the discovery of entirely new treatment methods. For the present, appropriate treatment of the elderly patient with a hematologic malignancy demands a thoughtful and careful physician.

Finally, we can contrast the primary cancer that is highly lethal but never metastasizes with its counterpart, the primary cancer that never kills but whose metastases always do. The former, which arises from brain tissue, is less common in the elderly than in the middle-aged. Survival has improved in recent years but there is room for much more. The latter type, that in which the primary tumor never kills, may be a bellwether in the development of sophistication of diagnosis and efficiency of chemotherapy. However, at present, an elderly patient with either one of these cancers deserves gentle and careful treatment.

In conclusion, the secrets of both aging and cancer, as well as of increased cancer with increased age, are probably locked deep in the nuclei of cells, perhaps in DNA itself. We may ultimately be able to devise more efficient methods of cancer treatment and these may well be made possible by advances in molecular biology. Until these improvements in understanding and therapy come however, we are best advised to keep in focus the finitude of human life and the natural histories of various kinds of cancers. Then, balancing benefit and risk to each patient, particularly the elderly, we will be better physicians.

Recent Results in Cancer Research

Sponsored by the Swiss League against Cancer. Editor in Chief: P. Rentchnick, Genève